THE TELEMENTAL HEALTH WORKBOOK

30+ Youth Friendly Activities for Mental Health Professionals

Flor Chaidez PPSC, LCSW
Veronica Obregon LCSW, Ed.D.

innovativeink
PUBLISHING
A Division of Kendall Hunt

innovativeink
PUBLISHING

www.innovativeinkpublishing.com
Send all inquiries to:
4050 Westmark Drive
Dubuque, IA 52004-1840

Print ISBN: 979-8-3851-6218-5
Ebook ISBN: 979-8-3851-6219-2

Published in the United States of America

Table of Contents

2024 Preface

Lessons Learned

In 2020, we authored our initial publication to support our colleagues—mental health providers—who successfully transitioned their organizations, agencies, and private practices to remote telemental health services (TMH). The global COVID-19 pandemic rapidly altered the landscape of mental health practice, necessitating this shift. Our aim was to synthesize academic research that underpinned this transition and to compile practical activities into a user-friendly manual for clinicians. We want to thank our readers for supporting our work and as we work to support mental health clinicians using telemental health.

Now, four years since the initial publication, we have expanded our work by adding more activities and providing a Spanish translation. The second edition includes 10 additional activities, offering clinicians a wider array of tools. The inclusion of a Spanish translation responds to the repeated requests from our readers and colleagues, who highlighted the scarcity of Spanish-language mental health resources. Our goal remains to bridge this gap, providing culturally relevant tools that resonate with clients' lived experiences.

Throughout this journey, we have gleaned valuable insights, and current research indicates both promising advantages and notable challenges in the implementation of telemental health services (Lipschitz et al., 2023). The necessity for culturally grounded tools in remote settings is evident, as telemental health has swiftly become integral to mental health services .

We have all learned some big lessons since 2020. The American Psychological Association's study on clinicians' perspectives revealed a demand for further training to ensure the delivery of high-quality remote mental health care (Lipschitz et al., 2023). The Advantages of Telemental Health seem to outweigh the disadvantages of remote work; which is why we continue to step up to provide resources for mental health clinicians. Table 1 below provides a review of the advantages listed in the research conducted by the American Psychological Association.

Table 1

Provider Perspectives on Telemental Health Implementation: Advantages	
Increased Utilization: TMH makes it easier for clients to show up to their sessions.	
Access	· Significantly improved patient access (eliminating the need for reliable transportation or childcare, avoiding traffic, saving on parking costs, and reducing health risks during the pandemic).
Attendance	· Reduction in no-shows, with some noting that TMH sessions were more likely to start on time. · Simplicity of turning on a computer was particularly helpful for clients who often struggled to arrive punctually for appointments
Therapeutic Process: Additional opportunities to build rapport.	
Clinical Insight	· Increased opportunities to build a rapport that was not possible in person because they were able to see where they lived and meet collateral contacts (family, friends, pets).
Self Disclosure	· Some clients were more willing to disclose sensitive topics through TMH and were even more willing to do so by telephone (issues to consider were diagnosis, age of client and technology challenges).
Provider Wellbeing: More time for personal life and control over workspace	
Work Life Balance	· Less time on commute to work, being able to take midday breaks to exercise or do chores contributed to work life harmony
Workplace Quality	· Home workspaces had a window or better air quality than their traditional office. · Participants who usually used office space reported that consistently working in a single location enhanced their clinical care due to easier access to materials such as books and handouts.

Note. For disadvantages, please review Lipschitz et al. (2023) for more information.

2020 Preface

This book was written to support mental health providers who have shifted to telemental health services as a result of COVID19, an environmental stressor, or a natural disaster. The COVID19 pandemic abruptly changed the face of American mental health in the middle of March 2020. Before that, most mental health providers and their clients had access to schools, community mental health settings and environments that were safe for face-to-face mental health support. February 29th, 2020 is the date of the first official COVID 19 death reported in the U.S. and the number quickly grew at an exponential pace (Worldometers.info, 2020). By March 15th there were 73 deaths that grew to 109,000 deaths by June 3, 2020 (Worldometers.info, 2020). March 15th also marked the first day of "Quarantine" in Los Angeles. COVID19 public health measures altered the shape of our culture by requiring most people in the country to shutter their doors as the calls for social distancing escalated. Mental health providers were considered essential workers, but most were unable to continue face-to-face contact and had to quickly shift to online mental health.

This shift or pivot to online environments was easy for most but challenging for many others who scrambled to find training and support. Clark and Estes (Clark, 2008) describe a gap analysis model to help understand why people do not perform their roles in job settings. They argue that it has to do with a motivation, knowledge, or tools/resources gap. Basically, people underperform because they don't want to do their job, they don't know how to do their job, or they don't have the tools and resources to do their best work. We hope that this workbook motivates mental health providers to want to engage in online mental health because the evidence base describes this as a promising and effective practice. This workbook will also provide tools for mental health providers to use to help them answer the question: What can I do online with my clients? This book provides tools that help mental health providers work with their clients as our community moves to online environments to improve access to treatment.

Promising Practice Evidence

Let's begin with the evidence. A simple Google Scholar search using the terms telemental health, telebehavioral health and virtual mental health reveals over 108,500 studies conducted between 2015 and 2020. Another Google Scholar search with the term "online mental health" reveals over 800,000 studies conducted between 2015-2020. This delivery model is well studied and researched and has been dissected in thousands of studies all over the world even before the COVID19 pandemic. Telemental health is not a new phenomenon. It is an evidence informed delivery method that has many applications not only to be used during quarantines. So don't give up on it yet!

In fact, this delivery method is here to stay and much of the evidence reports that it is effective (Hilty et al., 2013). The academic research points to very promising results in several domains for the use of telemental health (Hilty et al., 2013). Telemental health shows promise in providing access to services, providing support after natural disasters, trauma, caregiver support and ADHD to name a few.

Access

Telemental health improves access to mental health services for communities impacted by poverty, health and education disparities and immigration status. Telemental health services have been used to overcome barriers to referrals from primary care providers to mental health providers (Contreras et al., 2018; Myers & Comer, 2016). Telemental health services have also been used to provide access to rural populations who don't live near a mental health agency (Ulzen, Williamson, Foster, & Parris-Barnes, 2013). Given that the current and future quarantines impair a person's ability to leave their home, it is logical that mental health providers should learn how to provide telemental health to their clients to improve access.

Trauma

Telemental health has shown some promise and effectiveness in trauma work (Hassija & Gray, 2011; Jones et al., 2014; Stewart, Orengo-Aguayo, Cohen, Mannarino, & de Arellano, 2017; Stewart, Orengo-Aguayo, Wallace, Metzger, & Rheingold, 2019). Trauma informed mental health providers are aware that trauma is real, trauma affects cognition and affects brain development (Brunzell, Stokes, & Waters, 2016). Some research has shown that trauma-focused, cognitive–behavioral therapy (TF-CBT) via telemental health technology is an effective way to treat children and families (Jones et al., 2014).

Natural Disaster

Telemental health has also been used to support millions of people in the aftermath of natural disasters (Augusterfer, Ef, Mollica, & Lavelle, 2015; Augusterfer, Eugene, Mollica, & Lavelle, 2018; Revere et al., 2011). On March 13th, the US declared a nationwide emergency identifying the COVID19 Pandemic as a natural health disaster. Studies show effectiveness in working with victims of man-made disasters, wars, hurricanes, tsunamis and earthquakes (Augusterfer et al., 2015). Telemental health support can also critically reduce the negative psychological impact of disasters (Augusterfer et al., 2018).

Therapeutic Rapport

Telemental health may be a new direction for many clinicians, but it has been used for the past 20 years in different settings and with constantly evolving technologies. There was hesitation by many clinicians who argued that online mental health would "just not be the same" and would impair the therapeutic relationship. Let's be clear, it isn't the same, but it is still very helpful and you can still build therapeutic rapport within online conditions (Glueck, 2013; Goldstein & Glueck, 2016; Grady et al., 2011; Lopez, Schwenk, Schneck, Griffin, & Mishkind, 2019). Therapeutic Rapport is considered by some to be the most important element for behavioral change (Stamoulos et al., 2016). The research also reports that client improvement is related to the client and therapist's ability to relate to each other (Lambert & Barley, 2001). Fortunately, there is a wealth of evidence that shows that clinicians can build therapeutic rapport while using telemental health (Glueck, 2013). See Appendix A for a list of strategies.

Conclusion

This book was written to provide creative yet concrete ideas and activities for use, while providing telemental health services to your clients. The worksheets are intended to be used by qualified professionals within therapeutic situations. The clinician should use their own clinical training, conduct a full assessment of appropriateness of fit, take developmental stages into consideration and continuously assess amenability of activities for their clients. The worksheets can be used at various points in the group or individual therapeutic relationship. The worksheets can help in identifying points of focus and aid in assessment. You may use any activity in any order that you see fit or that you feel is appropriate for your client. You can choose any activity at your own professional discretion. It is assumed that you are practicing within the legal and ethical protocols of your mental health discipline.

Research shows that telemental health is a promising practice used in various settings and with diverse populations. The applications are endless. The book is organized to give you a review of the research that supports the use of telemental health, then provides 25 activities for you to use and ends with an appendix that provides relevant resources and handouts. The references page provides a rich list of readings and academic sources used to inform our arguments and intended for your further reading. We must include a disclaimer that this workbook does not replace or take the place of clinical supervision. Please stay within the scope of your practice and use your training and experience to assess the appropriateness of fit to diagnosis and developmental stages of your clients before you select any of these activities. We hope that you use and enjoy the activities we collected for you to spark your imagination and motivation to engage in Tele-mental health.

Contributions

We would like to express our heartfelt gratitude to the experts who contributed to our book. Their dedication and expertise in translation, creative illustration, and mental health expertise have been instrumental in bringing this workbook to life.

Guadalupe Solis provided professional translation services, helping us convert key sections of the text from English to Spanish. This was crucial for our readers who work with bilingual clients and needed resources that address the mental health needs of Spanish-speaking communities.

Frando Valentino, our talented illustrator, created user-friendly and replicable images for our handouts. His artistic vision added a visual charm that makes the workbook more engaging and accessible.

Jaqueline Ferrer, MSW collaborated with Flor Chaidez, LCSW to develop ten new activities for the book. Her invaluable creativity and hard work significantly enhanced the content, making it even more effective and enriching for our readers.

To each of these amazing individuals, we extend our deepest thanks. Your contributions have made a lasting impact on this project and the communities it will serve.

Activities

ALL AGES

Anxious Panda

Objectives:
- Provide psycho-education regarding somatic symptoms of anxiety.
- Build awareness regarding anxiety and bodily cues.

Supplies needed for clinician	**Supplies needed for client**
1. Handout	1. Handout

Instructions
1. Share questions on screen
2. Explore with client the various ways the panda is experiencing worry or anxiety
3. Clinician may also use this as a tool for conversation starter and not share screen with client.

Useful websites, tools, resources or notes:

ANXIOUS PANDA

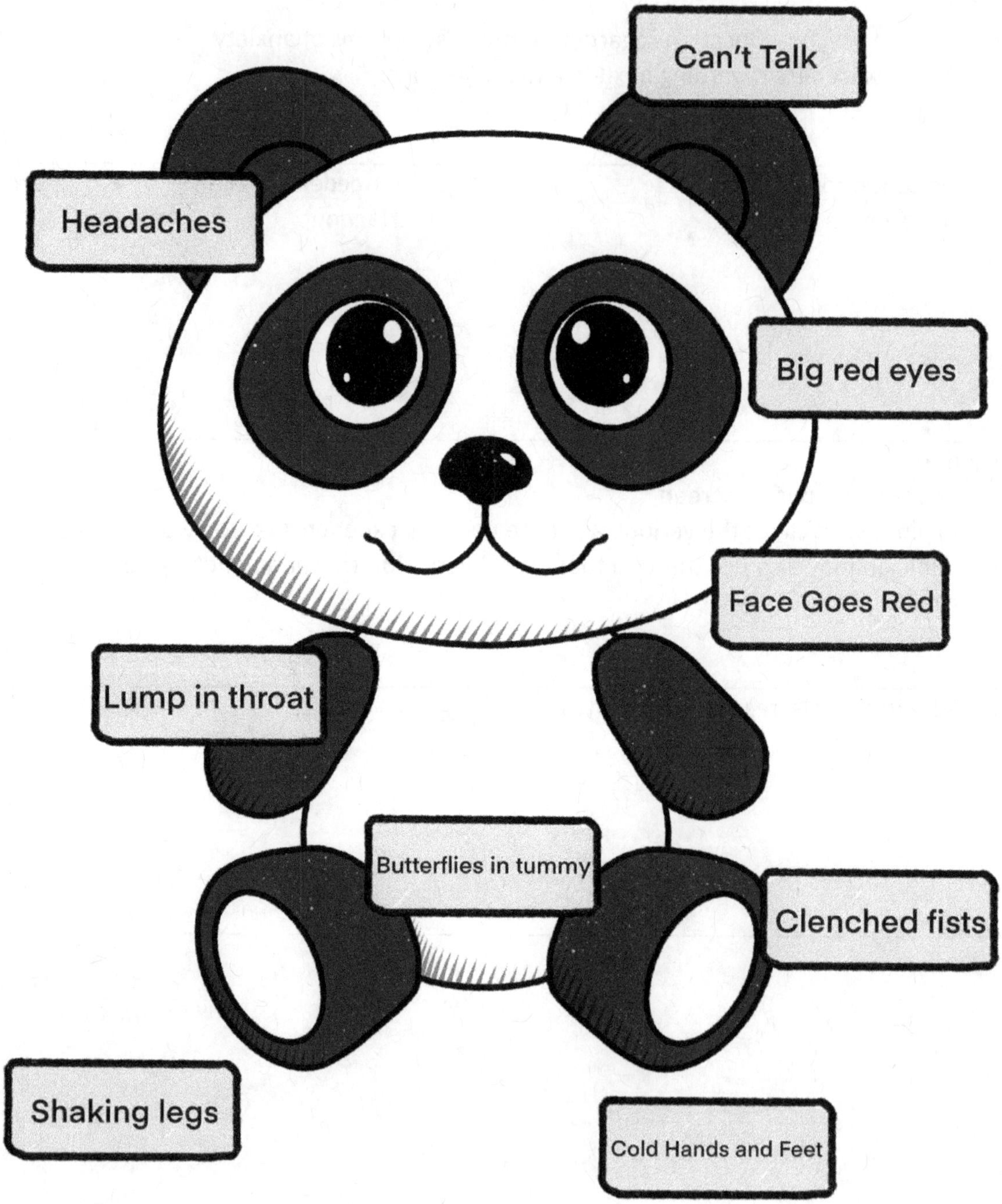

ALL AGES

Open Ended Questions

Objectives:

- To help clients articulate thoughts, feelings and emotions.
- To build therapeutic rapport.
- To help clients articulate thinking.
- Motivate clients to share relevant material about their life, way of thinking and beliefs.

Supplies needed for clinician	**Supplies needed for client**
2. Handout	2. Handout

Instructions

4. Share questions on screen
5. Ask client to pick what they want to answer by choosing a color.
6. Clinician may also use this as a tool for conversation starter and not share screen with client.

Useful websites, tools, resources or notes:

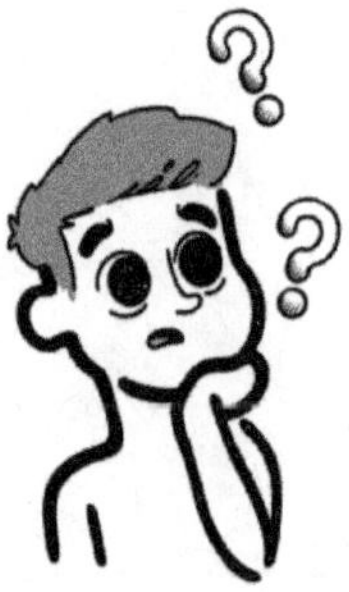

Open Ended Questions

What was your favorite part of the day?	What do You like about school?	How are you planning to do that?
What make a nice Friend?	What are you excited about this week?	What could you have done instead?
If you could have a magic power what would it be ?	What do you like most about the weekend? Why?	What is your favorite day of the week?
If you could travel anywhere where would it be?	What is your favorite movie?	What is your favorite book?
What does this remind you of? Why?	How does it work?	How did that happen?
How can you make things better?	How are these the Same/ Different?	How do you feel about what happened?
What Choice would you have made?	How can you make that person feel better?	What do you love most about your family?

ALL AGES

Breaking Down Anger

Objectives:
- Explore what thoughts, feelings, or memories are behind the anger.
- Teach client that that beneath anger can be varying emotions that lead to the demonstration of anger.
- Provide a visual metaphor of what it means when you say "behind the anger".

Supplies needed for clinician	**Supplies needed for client**
1. Handout	1. Handout 2. Pencil/Pen

Instructions
1. Introduce worksheet to the client
2. Share your screen or email to client.
3. Discuss the emotion of anger and what lies beneath the client's expression of anger and what circumstances may have triggered emotion.
4. Tell client to circle and list as many things that they can think of that happened, what they thought, what they remembered before becoming angry.
    a. Give an example.

Useful websites, tools, or resources:

Sometimes on the surface it looks like anger……

- What you see on the surface is only a small part of what is hidden underneath.
- But you may be feeling sadness, offended, annoyed, jealous, rejected, grief, embarrassment, hungry, overwhelmed, hurt, stressed, anxious……
- Think about what has brought about your anger?

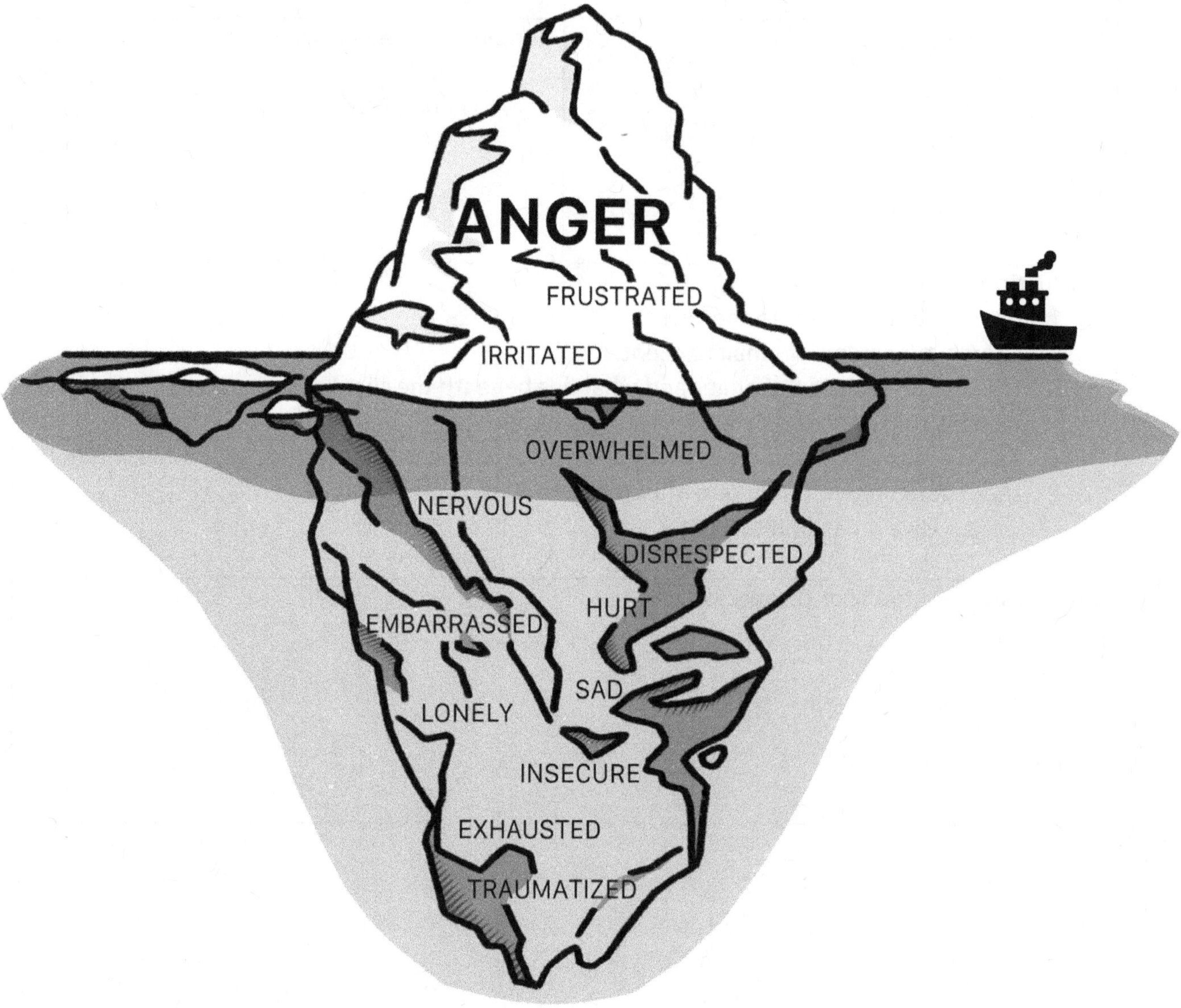

ALL AGES

Gratitude Exercise

Objectives:

- Reframing exercise to move from feeling without to feeling abundant.
- Increase positive emotions and introduction to mindfulness.

Supplies needed for clinician	**Supplies needed for client**
1. Handout	1. Handout 2. Something to write 3. Notepad to take notes if not using handout.

Instructions:

1. Introduce the concept of being thankful- gratitude and benefits. (See Greater Good Science Center Link.)
2. Share worksheet with client (email, text or share screen).
3. You can use writing tool to write client answers.
4. Client my also share responses in chat box.
5. Gratitude exercise can be done intermittently or introduced as a daily exercise that client can practice as mindfulness.

Useful websites, tools, resources or notes:

The Greater Good Science Center studies the psychology, sociology, and neuroscience of well-being and teaches skills that foster a thriving, resilient, and compassionate society
https://ggsc.berkeley.edu

START AND END EACH DAY WITH A GRATEFUL HEART

Things I like about being me

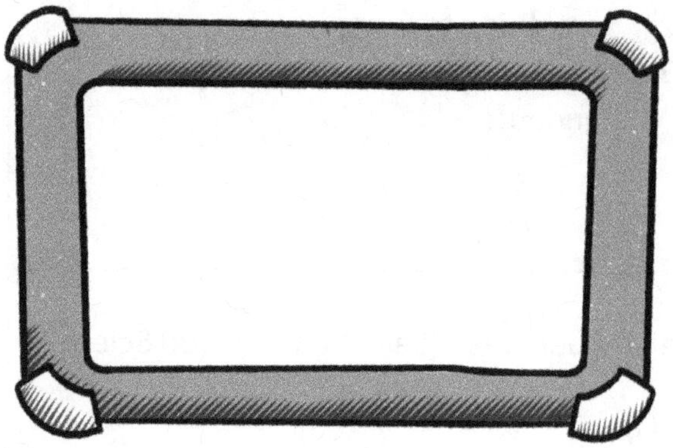

I am thankful for these People

What went well today

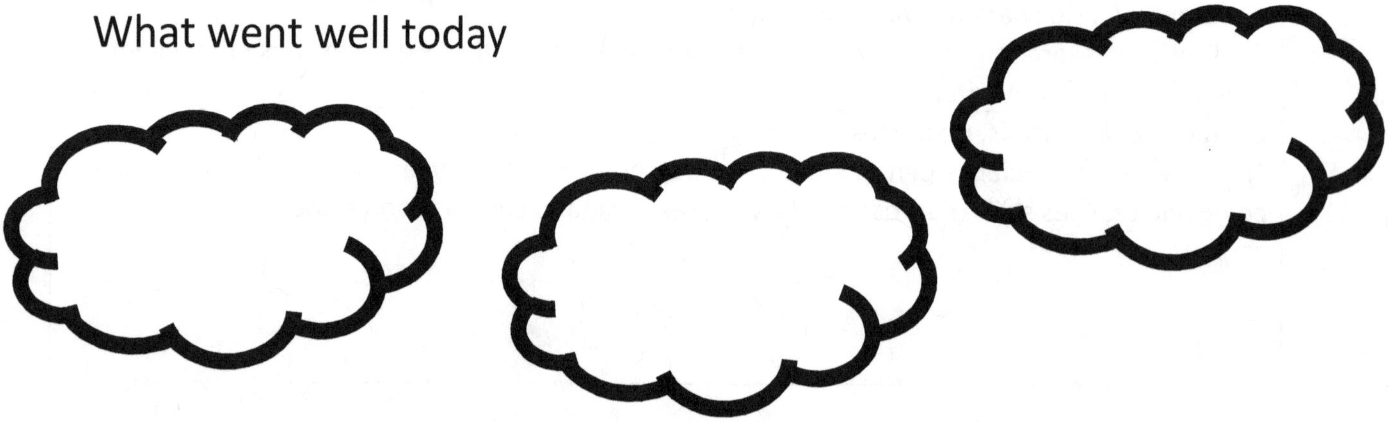

I am Thankful for

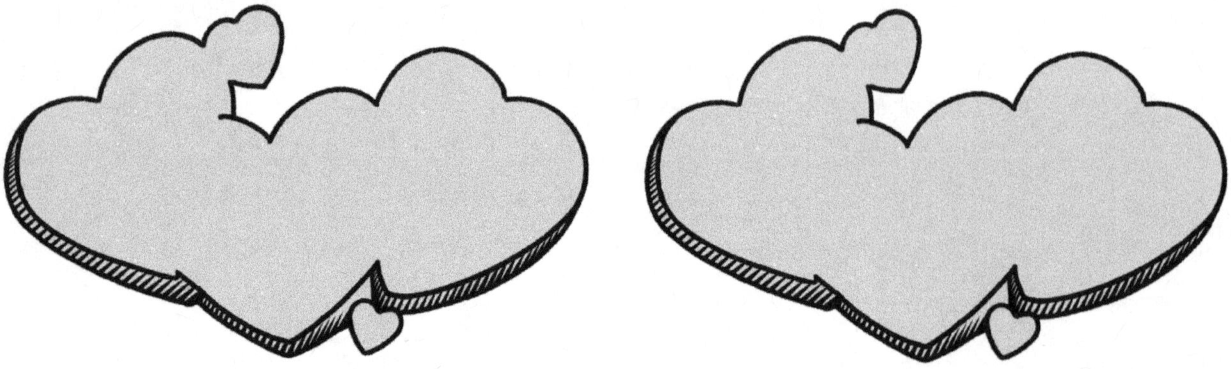

ALL AGES

Getting to Know You

Objectives:

- To familiarize yourself with the client.
- To build therapeutic rapport.
- To gather identifying information for ongoing assessment.

Supplies needed for clinician	**Supplies needed for client**
1. Handout	1. Handout 2. Pencil/Pen 3. Notepad to take notes if not using handout.

Instructions:

Clinician to introduce worksheet to client by sharing teleconference screen. You may allow client to pick which questions they may want to answer. This worksheet may be spread over several sessions. If client is younger, clinician may choose questions. Depending on what you may be, treating client for, clinician may be intentional about information gathering.

Useful websites, tools, or notes:

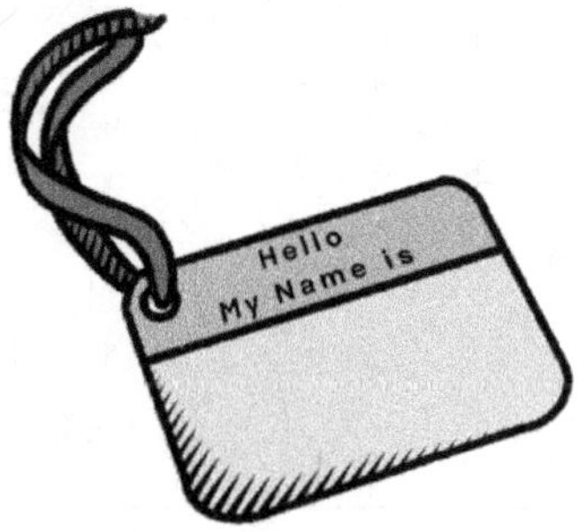

GETTING TO KNOW YOU

I like to ______________________________

I'm good at______________________________

My friends say ______________________________

I worry when ______________________________

One word that described me is ______________________________

I get angry when ______________________________

My family is ______________________________

I get upset when______________________________

I become sad when ______________________________

I am afraid of ______________________________

I wish ______________________________

When I grow up I want to be ______________________________

In ten years from now I want ______________________________

My Favorite Thing to do is ______________________________

I love ______________________________

I hate ______________________________

I once had a dream about ______________________________

ALL AGES

Feeling Identification

Objectives

- Assist client in exploring different types of feelings.
- Learning to name the feeling associated with behavior.
- Build therapeutic relationship by providing positive regard.
- Provide psychoeducation about empathy/compassion.

Supplies needed for clinician	Supplies needed for client
1. Handout	1. Handout 2. Pencil/Pen 3. Notepad to take notes if not using handout.

Instructions

1. Introduce concept of "feelings" with the client. (see website)
2. Share worksheet with the client using email, text or share screen.
3. Older client may want to choose which questions they want to answer.
4. Younger children may need to be read the questions.
    a. Client does not have to answer all questions in one session.

Useful websites, tools, resources or notes

- Difference between feelings and emotions: https://www.psychologytoday.com/us/blog/hide-and-seek/201412/whats-the-difference-between-feeling-and-emotion
- This worksheet is a useful precursor to the CBT worksheet.

FEELING IDENTIFICATION ACTIVITY

Please write down or describe the following

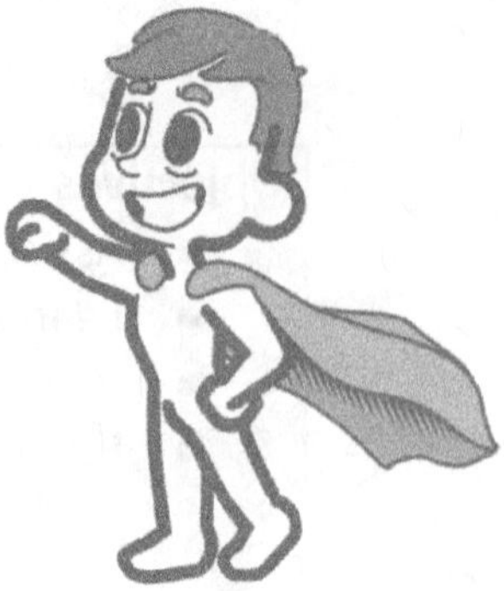

- A time you felt scared:
- A time you felt sad:
- A time you felt happy:
- A time you felt angry:
- A time you felt proud of yourself:
- A time you felt you had no control:
- Something you are afraid of:
- What you think/ feel when you think about yourself:
- What you think/ feel what do you think about your mom:
- What you think/ feel when you think about your dad:
- What you think/ feel when you think about your friends:
- What would you describe your school as:
- Something you wish you could do over again:
- What would you do with a million dollars?
- Three things you like about yourself:
- 3 things you wish you could change or don't like about yourself:
- Three things you would like to do before you die:
- Something you would like to change in your life:
- What is a strength that you have? When was the last time you were able to use your strength to change a negative situation into a positive one?
- How you felt while doing this exercise:

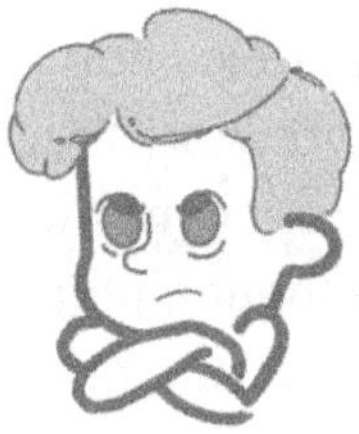

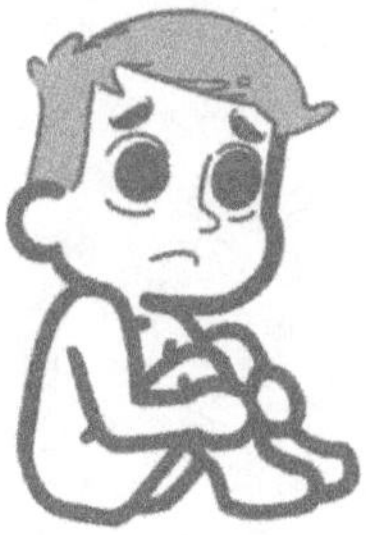

ALL AGES

Emotions Charades

Objectives

- Practice emotions and feeling identification
- Assist with correcting hurtful past narratives.
- Build therapeutic relationship by having client move out of their comfort zone.

Supplies needed for clinician	**Supplies needed for client**
1. Handout	1. Handout 2. Something to write 3. Notepad to take notes if not using handout.

Instructions

1. Introduce the game of charades to client. Tell client to choose a phrase then the player must act out the charade while the other player has 3 minutes to guess the correct answer. If they get it correct within the time limit, the team scores a point. The clinician is one team and the client is another. They both takes their turns and this continues until all of the ideas are used up. The team with the most points wins. You can decide to play up to a certain score or set a time limit for the game.
2. Share worksheet with the client by email, text or sharing screen.
3. Older client may want to choose what they role-play and younger children may need suggestions.
4. Client may need guidance and encouragement from clinician.
5. Use as a tool for gaining a better understanding of client's internal processes as well as recounting past narratives. Best if used in middle of therapeutic relationship when there is high attunement.

Useful websites, tools, or resources:

EMOTIONS CHARADES

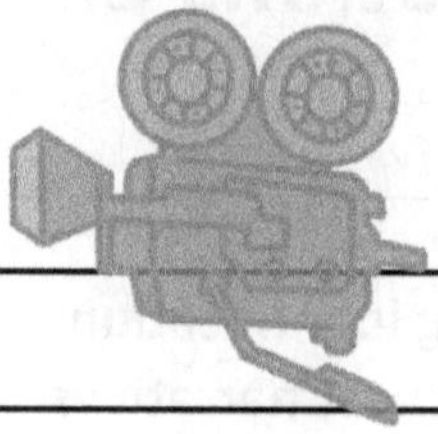

Going on a rollercoaster
Scoring a goal
Your sister breaking your favorite toy
Eating broccoli
Getting straight A’s
Breaking your neighbors window
Making Presentation in front of class
Not getting invited to a friend’s birthday party
Falling of your bike
Your mom being upset with you
Your ipad/ cell phone being taken away
You win the spelling bee
You scored the winning goal for your team
You are going to have a new baby brother or sister
You are going to family birthday party
It’s Christmas morning

ALL AGES

Coping Skills Exercise

Objectives	
• Psychoeducation about ineffective/ hurtful coping vs. effective/healthy. • Build coping skills and protective factors.	
Supplies needed for clinician	**Supplies needed for client**
1. Handout	1. Handout 2. Pencil/Pen 3. Notepad to take notes if not using handout.

Instructions

1. Introduce worksheet to the client
2. Share screen, email or text client.
3. Ask client to read from two columns and make their own "good" and "bad" list.
    a. Client may need guidance and prompting from clinician.

Useful websites, tools, resources or notes

Use processing questions at the bottom of page to elaborate on client's coping skills. Use as a guide to make goals for positive coping and as a toolbox for client.

- What are some of your good coping skills?
- How can you turn some of your poor coping skills into better habits?
- Can you think of any others?

COPING SKILLS EXERCISE

How we handle stressful situations can affect how we feel. There are good coping and bad coping skills. Sometimes coping skills can become habits.

**Make two columns on a sheet of paper and put each of the coping skills under good or bad

Sleep all day	Take a bath or a shower
Coloring	Talk to my parents
Watch TV	Read a book, comic, or magazine
Call a friend	Yell and scream
Eat a snack	Punch a pillow
Put on a nice outfit	Leave the room
Do jumping jacks	Spend time outside
Crumple/ rip up paper	Throw things
Smell something nice (lavender)	Squeeze an ice cube
Snap a rubber band	Cover/ close your eyes
Take deep breaths	Hurt yourself
Crush soda cans	Say curse words
Clench your fists	Play with a pet
Dance	Cook something
Cry	Count to ten
Talk to my therapist	Hurt someone
Sing	Do a puzzle
Draw	Crush cardboard boxes
Stretch	Yell into a pillow
Drinking water	Put on lotion
Positive self- talk	Give yourself a hug
Play a board game	Tidy up
Hug a stuffed animal	Speak with a Friend

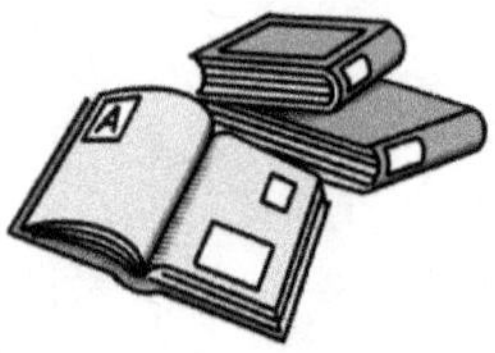

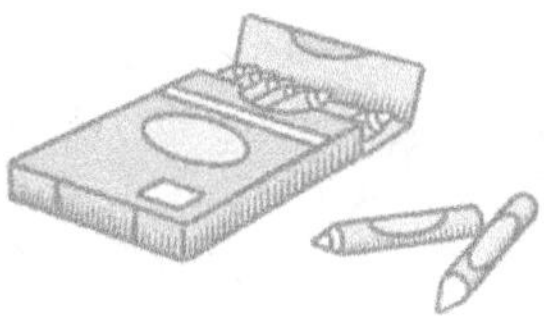

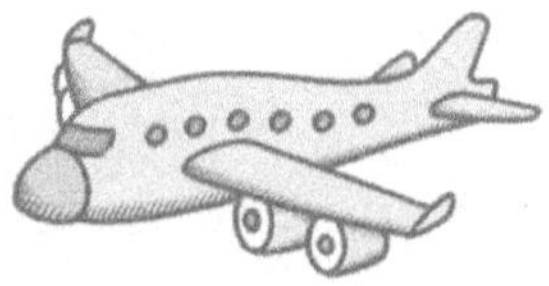

ALL AGES

CBT Triangle

Objectives

- Help client make a connection between thoughts, feelings and behaviors.
- Learn to recognize distorted thinking.
- Learn to reframe distorted thinking.

Supplies needed for clinician	**Supplies needed for client**
1. Handout	1. Handout 2. Pencil/Pen 3. Notepad to take notes if not using handout.

Instructions

1. Clinician to introduce concept of the relationship between thoughts, feelings and actions
2. Share screen, email or text client.
3. The worksheet aids in visualization of concept and client can also read prompts. Use prompts on bottom of page to facilitate with exploration of concept. "Hot" thoughts refer to mad or angry thoughts and "warm" thoughts refer to positive or calm thoughts.

Useful websites, tools, resources or notes:

CBT TRIANGLE

It's All Related

Sometimes we have "hot" thoughts... What color might that be? What Feelings might you be feeling? What Actions might you take?

What about if you were feeling "warm" thoughts... What color might that be? What feelings might you be feeling? What Actions might you take?
We have many thoughts throughout the day, sometimes we act on them, sometimes not... Take a minute to ask yourself... what am I feeling?, how is it making me think?, how am I behaving?

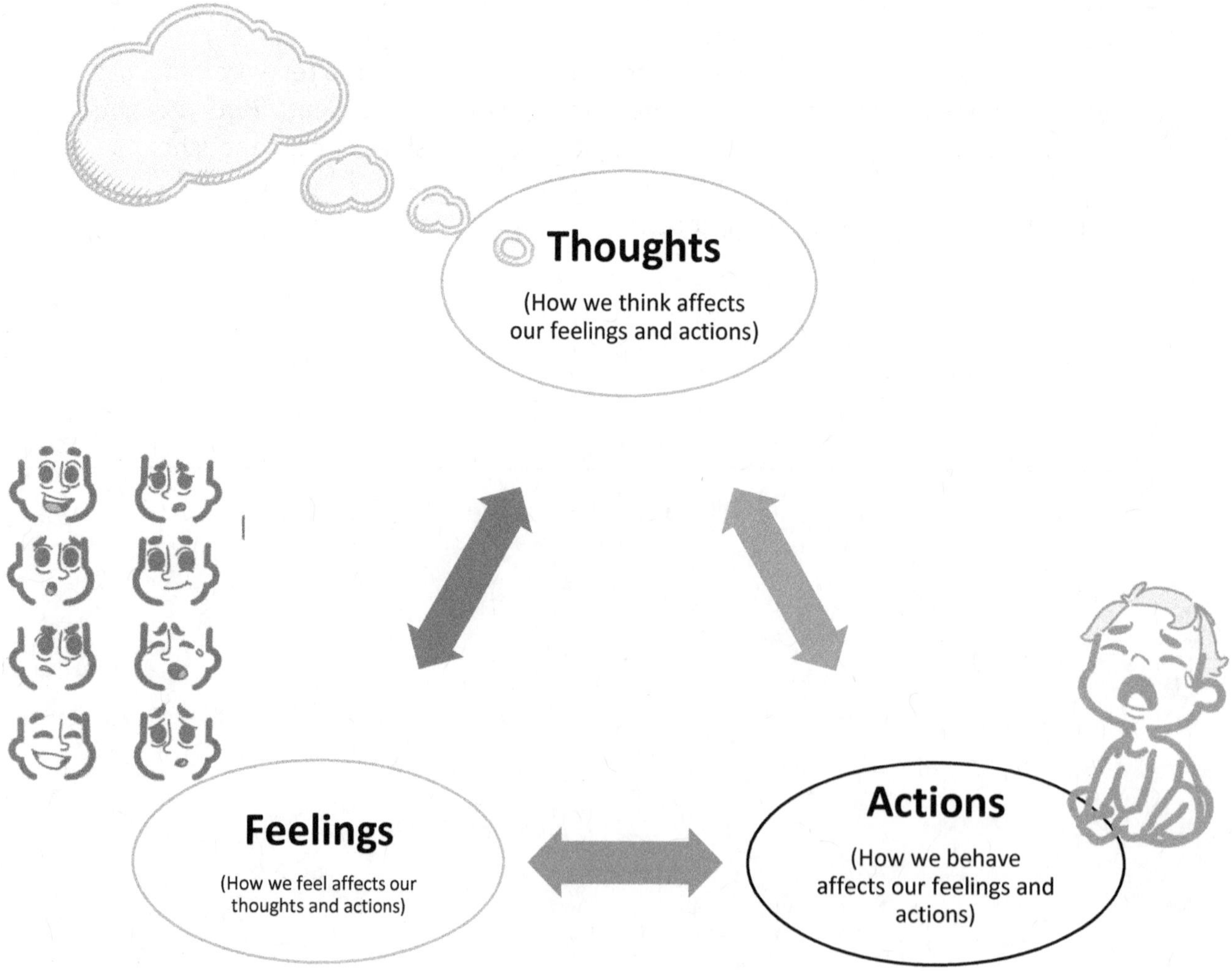

CHILDREN
5+

Online Scavenger Hunt

Objectives	
• Build therapeutic relationship. • Encourages rapport by using prompts as an opportunity to process difficult feelings and promote positive coping.	
Supplies needed for clinician 1. Handout	**Supplies needed for client** 1. Handout 2. Pencil/Pen 3. Notepad to take notes if not using handout.
Instructions: 1. Introduce worksheet to the client 2. Share screen, email or text client. 3. Go through list in any order	
Useful websites, tools, resources or notes: It is a fun way to get to know your client. Follow with elaboration questions that include: • Why is that your favorite color? • How come that makes you laugh? • What is your favorite memory with your favorite toy?	

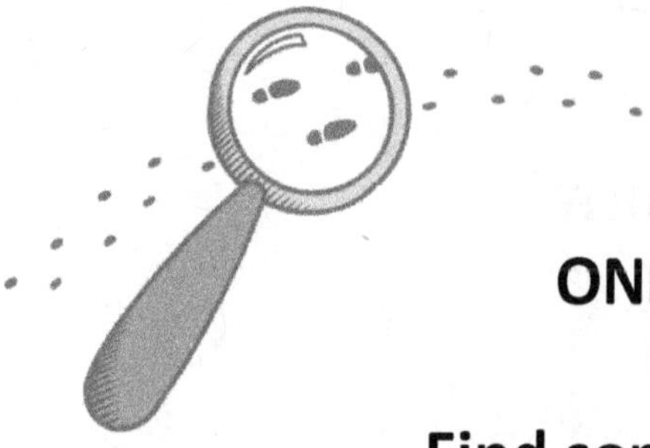

ONLINE SCAVENGER HUNT

Find something in your home that...

- Is your Favorite color
- You enjoy looking at
- Makes you laugh
- Makes you feel safe
- Is your favorite toy
- You like to do for fun
- You are proud of
- Is unique
- Brings you comfort
- Is your favorite picture
- Brings back a happy memory
- You use to calm yourself down if you are upset or angry
- Reminds you of someone you miss right now
- Is your favorite snack
- Is your choice

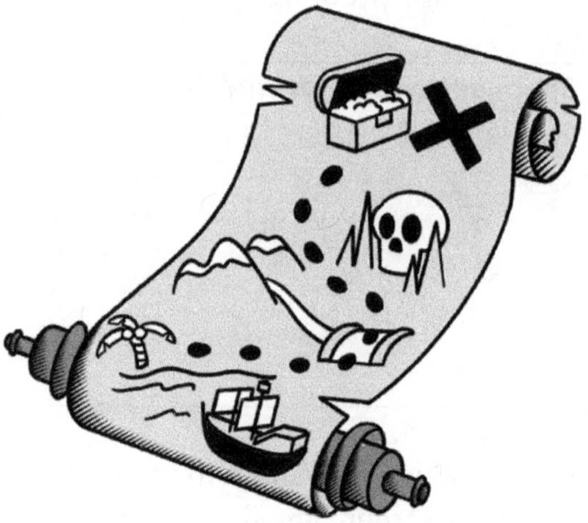

CHILDREN
5+

A Journal About Me

Objectives
- Model the importance of reflection.
- Help to organize thoughts/ executive functioning.
- Encourage as a positive coping skill.

Supplies needed for clinician	Supplies needed for client
1. Handout	1. Handout 2. Pencil/Pen 3. Notepad to take notes if not using handout.

Instructions
1. Introduce the game to the client
2. Share screen, email or text client
    a. This aids in visualization of game and client can also read prompts.
3. Use writing tool on video platform to write in clients answers
4. Or, depending on clients age, have them write in chat box or on handout

Useful websites, tools, resources or notes:

A Journal About Me ...

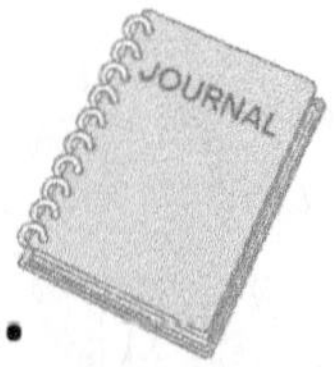

Written and illustrated by:	
DRAW A PICTURE OF YOURSELF	
8 Things that I Love	
1.	5
2.	6.
3.	7.
4.	8
Favorite	
Animal	Movie
Food	Friend
Color	Place
What Happened On	
Monday	
Tuesday	
Wednesday	
Thursday	
Friday	
Saturday	
Sunday	

ALL AGES

Behavior Chart

Objectives • Helps parents monitor child's behavior. • Helps parent reinforce positive behavior. • Helps parent refocus on client's positive vs. negative behavior.	
Supplies needed for clinician 1. Handout	**Supplies needed for client** 1. Handout 2. Pencil/Pen 3. Notepad to take notes if not using handout.
Instructions 1. Explain the chart to the parent and the child 2. Parent tells child that they will assign Points--Certain number of points allows child/adolescent to get a reward/privilege Privileges and rewards are defined by child/adolescent and adult before beginning point chart. 3. Facilitate a discussion between parent and child to identify privileges and rewards 4. Number of points needed to gain a privilege is discussed before beginning point chart. a. It is important to begin with 2 to 3 behaviors and increase with 1 behavior after success of initial behaviors. b. Share behavior chart on the screen, assist parent in developing a behavior plan. Send to parent and monitor weekly. Encourage consistency.	
Useful websites, tools, resources or notes	

ALL AGES

BEHAVIOR CHART

CHORE/BEHAVIOR	POINTS
Brush Teeth	
Make Bed	
Clean up toys after use	
Read for 30 minutes	
Complete homework	
Clean room--be specific	
Take out garbage	
Wash dishes	
Set table	
Show respect--be specific	
Attend school daily	
Tell the truth	
Show politeness	
Receive good report/reports card from school	

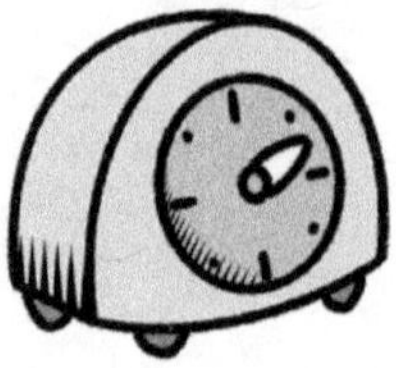

ALL AGES

Child Relaxation Script

Objectives
- Decrease the effects of stress on your mind and body.
- Teach a relaxation technique to cope with everyday stress along with stress related to various health problems.
- Teach a positive coping skill and increase protective factors.

Supplies needed for clinician	**Supplies needed for client**
1. Handout	1. Handout 2. Pencil/Pen 3. Notepad to take notes if not using handout.

Instructions
1. Introduce the concept of relaxation and meditation along with "quieting the mind".
2. Share a screen with client that is of a peaceful setting. For example, an ocean, meadow, nature, when you are introducing concept.
3. Ask client to turn their chair, but continue listening, and maybe close their eyes.
4. Familiarize yourself with script before reading it to client and follow processing questions at the bottom of page.

Useful websites, tools, resources or notes:
- Practice the script so it sounds natural and soothing to client.
- Sky scene that you can screen share: https://www.youtube.com/watch?v=cPtWBNQ83EM
- Processing Questions:
    - How did the activity make you feel
    - What did you like best? Least?
    - How could you use this activity?
    - What are the benefits?

CHILD SCRIPT

In a few minutes, I am going to say some things that I hope will help
You create a picture in your mind...
I am also going to ask you to relax different parts of your body.
Learning to relax will help you cope with angry, sad, and scary feelings
Find a comfortable position in your chair, not touching anyone,
In addition, take in a few relaxing breaths...
Close your eyes and relax...
Wiggle a little bit and make yourself comfortable...
Alright, take a few more relaxing breaths...
Breathe in ... breathe out...breathe in... and breathe out.
That's it – you are feeling peaceful.
If you were angry, you can picture yourself moving from hot to cold on the thermometer.
Becoming more and more relaxed, cold, peaceful.
Now, with your eyes closed, pretend that you are on
A white fluffy cloud, high in the sky on a beautiful day
You are floating peacefully on that white fluffy cloud
Moving very slowly... you are as light as a feather...
And the fluffy cloud holds you safely... floating across the sky.
Now, as I count from 1 to 3, imagine that you are sinking deeper and deeper into the cloud... so the cloud is all around you
1...2...3
You are enjoying the ride on the cloud.
Now, notice your toes and feet, how relaxed they feel...
Notice your legs... all the muscles in your legs are light
And relaxed on the cloud. Notice your arms...
Notice your neck... notice your head...
Now you are very relaxed ... floating on the fluffy cloud...
Whenever you need to calm down and relax...Whenever you need to cool off... move from hot to cool on the thermometer.
Now, we are getting ready to stop our ride on the cloud. We will stop on the count of three...1...2...3
Open your eyes and stretch a little.

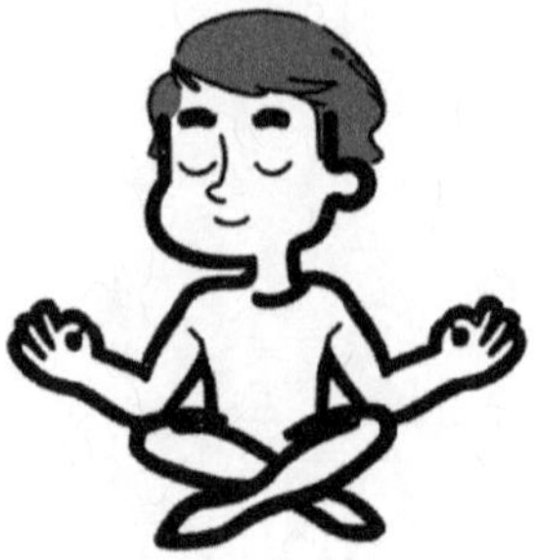

Children

Flipped My Lid Dice Game

Objectives:	
• To assist client in identifying triggers for their anger and exploring alternative ways of managing upsetting moments. • Increase positive coping skills.	
Supplies needed for clinician 1. Handout 2. Dice	**Supplies needed for client** 1. Handout 2. Pencil/Pen 3. Notepad to take notes if not using handout. 4. Dice
Instructions: 1. Introduce the game to the client 2. Share screen, email or text client a. This aids in visualization of game and client can also read prompts.	
Useful websites, tools, or resources:	

I’ve “Flipped my Lid” Dice Game

When I roll 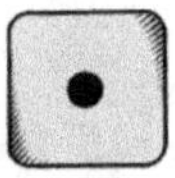 say one that makes you mad

When I roll 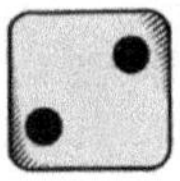 say one thing that you did to cool off after you were mad

When I roll 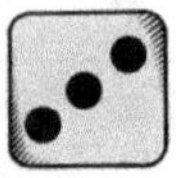 say one way you remained calm at school

When I roll 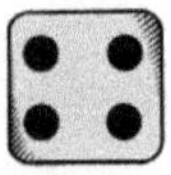 describe a time when you lost control

When I roll 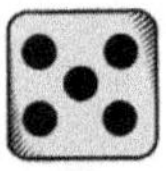 say how you felt after you were angry

When I roll 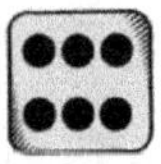 describe when you can do next time you become upset.

Children

Animal in You

Objectives ● Explore human traits and personality. ● Explore strengths-based traits.	
Supplies needed for clinician 1. Instructions Handout	**Supplies needed for client** 1. Instructions Handout 2. Pencil/Pen 3. Notepad to take notes if not using handout. 4. Paper, markers, colored pencils.
Instructions: 1. Ask client to draw an animal that they feel closely related to. 2. Ask client what characteristics they seen in that animal that are also related to themselves. a. Process with client how these attributes may be as source of strength within the client.	
Useful websites, tools, resources and notes:	

Animal In Me

All Ages

Feeling Colors

Objectives

- Help client identify and articulate emotions.
- Assist client in visualizing and describing abstract concepts of emotion.

Supplies needed for clinician	**Supplies needed for client**
1. Handout	1. Handout 2. Paper 3. Markers 4. Colored pencils.

Instructions

1. Introduce concept of colors as having certain feelings.
2. Have the client choose a color that describes how they are feeling today.
3. Have the client explain why this color is the best explanation of the feeling.
4. If in a group setting, find someone who chose the same color, and compare and contrast your reasons.
5. Ask client to share his work.

Useful websites, tools, resources and notes:
https://www.verywellmind.com/color-psychology-2795824

Feeling Colors

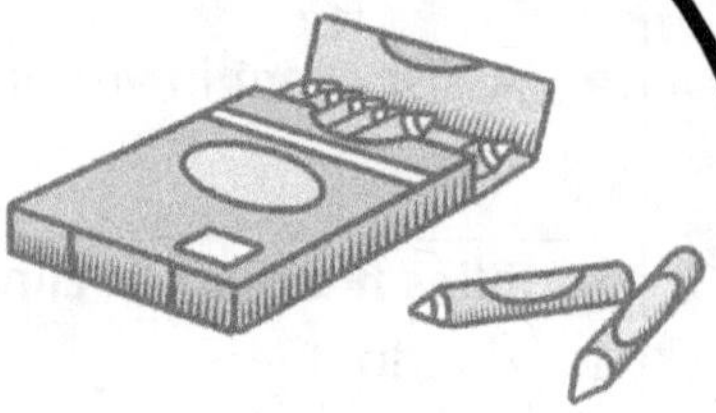

All Ages

Heartfelt Feelings

Objectives

- To help client process difficult emotions, situations and events.
- To visually express emotions.

Supplies needed for clinician	Supplies needed for client
1. Handout	1. Handout 2. Paper 3. Markers 4. Colored pencils

Instructions

1. Ask the client to color the heart to represent the emotions they are currently feeling.
    a. Processing question “How much are you feeling this?”
2. Adolescent clients: Ask client to write in what is in their heart.
    a. You can discuss the client's current well-being and any difficult feelings they may be experiencing.

Useful websites, tools, resources or notes:

HEART FELT FEELINGS

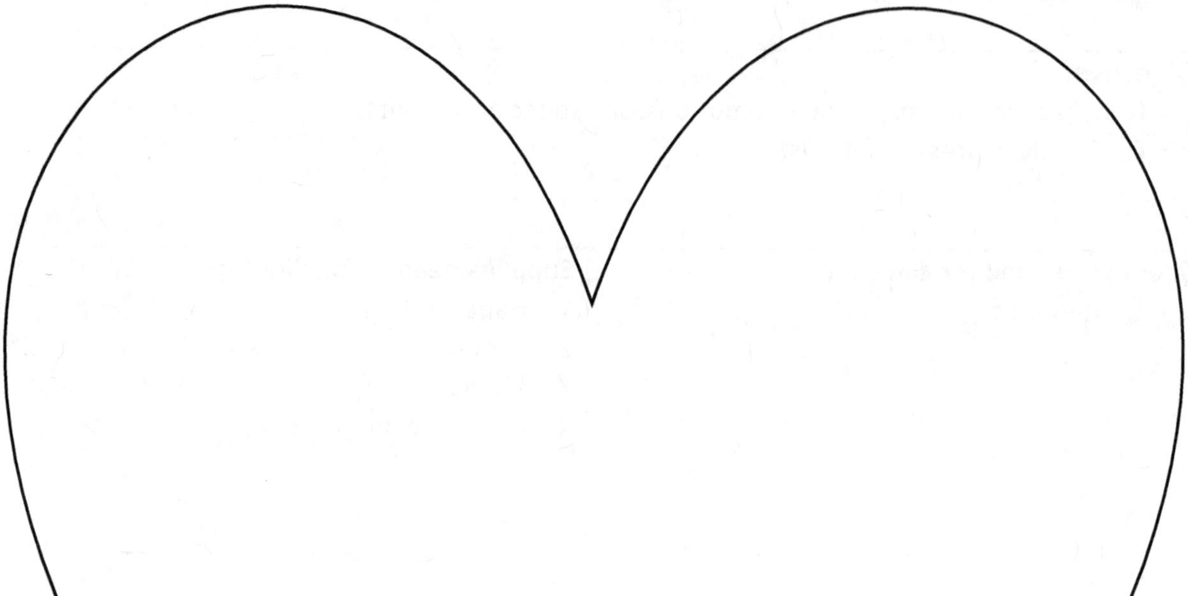

All Ages

Letter to Future Self

Objectives

- To motivate and work towards goals.
- Attain a future oriented perspective.
- To inspire hope.

Supplies needed for clinician	**Supplies needed for client**
1. Handout	1. Handout 2. Paper for notes 3. Pencil/Pen

Instructions:

1. Introduce the client to the concept of visualization.
2. Ask client to write a letter to their future self for either academic or personal goals.
3. The letter can have a 6-month time-line, school year, or birthday, opening date.

**My daughter wrote a letter when she was six and had me hold it until she was 18 , she recently opened it and it was very touching.

Useful websites, tools, resources or notes:

LETTER TO SELF

High School

'My Life' Music Playlist

(No Handout needed)

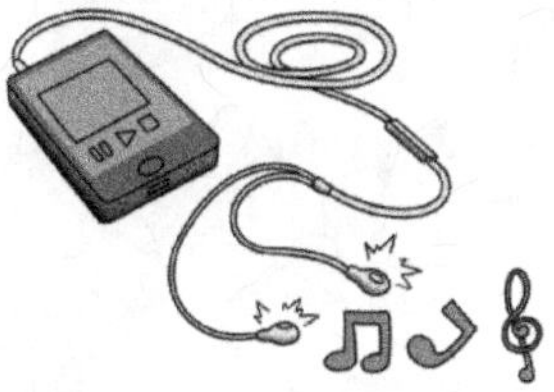

Objectives

- Identify and articulate emotions through music.
- Assist client in visualizing and describing abstract concept of emotion.
- Reflect and communicate through music.

Supplies needed for clinician	Supplies needed for client
1. Access to Spotify, Pandora, iTunes, You Tube or any other music app	1. Pencil/Pen 2. Access to Spotify, Pandora, iTunes, You Tube or any other music app

Instructions

1. Ask client create a playlist of their life using three to five songs.
2. Have client showcase one chapter of their life or their whole life. Have them explain what each song means to them.
    a. Why are these songs special?

Can also be used as a brain break.

Useful websites, tools, or resources:
https://www.psychologytoday.com/us/therapy-types/music-therapy

Children

Playdough Monster

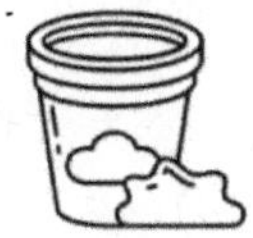

(No Handout needed)

Objectives:

- To process difficult emotions, situations and events.

Supplies needed for clinician	Supplies needed for client
1. Handout 2. Playdough	1. Playdough

Instructions

1. Ask client to create a "monster" with the playdough.
2. Discuss how monsters make them feel, how they might be able to overcome the monster and then have fun squishing the monster.
   - Can be a stress monster, worry monster, mean monster…etc
2. Join client in creating "monster" to assist with joining process.

Useful websites, tools, resources or notes:

- Playing with playdough also helps with attention and relieving stress.

Children

Puppets

(No Handout needed)

Objectives

- Work through situations, events, issues that are a concern to client or a pattern of behavior.

Supplies needed for clinician	Supplies needed for client
1. Handout	1. Paper lunch bags or socks 2. Markers or colored pencils 3. Glue

Instructions

1. Ask client to create their own puppet that represents themselves
2. Then ask client to act out a scene at the lunch table, or scenario of their choice, (possibly one that is causing them distress) pretending to be themselves.
3. Mental Health Provider encourages authenticity of performance, and gauges to see how clients perceive themselves as behaving, versus how they behave in reality.
4. Provider can also make their own puppet and engage in role-play.

Useful websites, tools, resources or notes:

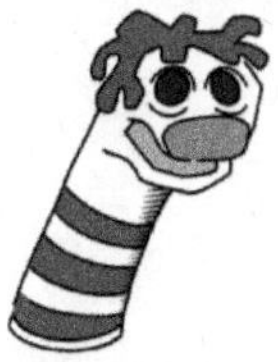

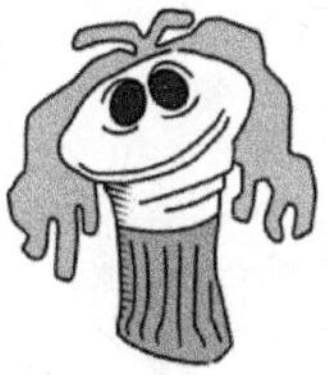

Children

Simon Says

(No Handout needed)

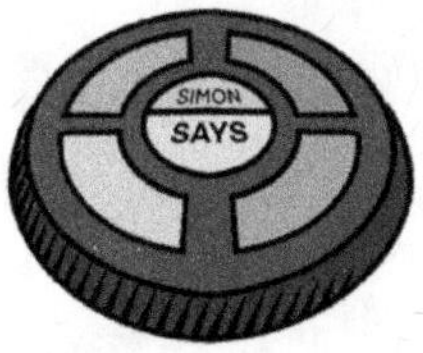

Objectives:

- To build therapeutic rapport.
- Work on listening skills and stimulus control.
- To engage in a brain-break activity.

Supplies needed for clinician	Supplies needed for client
1. Handout	

Instructions

1. One player is Simon and gives commands to client or group.
2. If they say "Simon says...sit down/ hop" everyone must do that action.
3. If they say just "sit down/ hop" everyone must remain still or they are out of the game.
4. Give directions with top- half of body if video only shows top half of your body.
   a. For example, "scratch your nose with right finger, pull your right ear with left hand, snap fingers, show jazz hands".... Accrue points for the directions received correctly.

Useful websites, tools, resources or notes:

Children

Online Madlibs

(No Handout Needed)

Objectives:

- Build client rapport.
- Enhance therapeutic relationship.
- Increase coping skills.

Supplies needed for clinician

1. Handout

Supplies needed for client

1. Handout
2. Pencil/Pen
3. Notepad to take notes if not using handout.
4. Dice

Instructions:

Explain how madlibs works. Log onto https://www.glowwordbooks.com/blog/category/kids-online-mad-libs/

Share teleconference screen with client. Engage student in creating silly humorous stories. Can be used as a brain break, reward or relationship builder.

Useful websites, tools;

https://www.glowwordbooks.com/blog/category/kids-online-mad-libs/

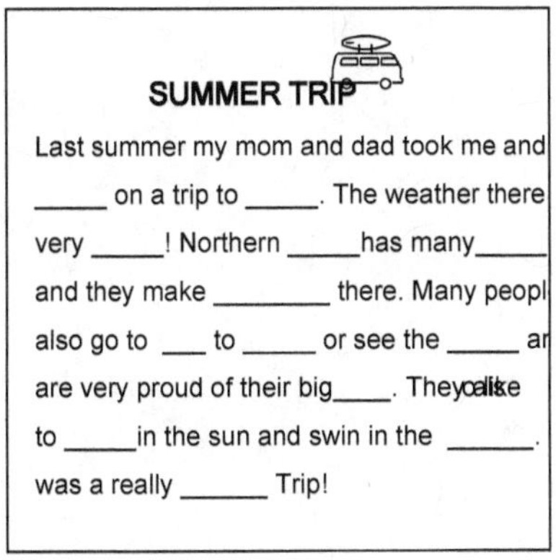

SUMMER TRIP

Last summer my mom and dad took me and
_____ on a trip to _____. The weather there
very _____! Northern _____has many_____
and they make ________ there. Many peopl
also go to ___ to _____ or see the _____ ar
are very proud of their big____. They alike
to _____in the sun and swin in the ______.
was a really ______ Trip!

All AGES

Goodbye Letter

<table>
<tr><td colspan="2">Objectives
• To help client articulate thoughts and feelings about grief.
• To help uncover difficulty thoughts and emotions related to the death of a loved one.</td></tr>
<tr><td>Supplies needed for clinician
1. Handout</td><td>Supplies needed for client
1. Handout
2. Pencil/Pen
3. Notepad to take notes if not using handout.</td></tr>
<tr><td colspan="2">Instructions
1. Share letter through email, text or on screen.
2. Provide client with sentence prompts to spark thinking
a. Have them complete the letter in session or as homework
3. Process any difficult emotions with client after letter.</td></tr>
<tr><td colspan="2">Useful websites, tools, resources or notes:
Consider ending with a 2-3 minute meditation.</td></tr>
</table>

I Will Miss You

To____________________________

I remember when

____

____

____

When you died I felt

____

____

____

What I will miss most about you is

____

____

____

Something you taught me

____

____

____

Thank you for

____

____

____

Love,

____

All AGES

Positive Self Talk

Objectives

- Assist client in building self-esteem and reframe negative thoughts.
- Helps reframe the way you look at stressful situations.
- Strength-based exercise, which also helps, build relationship with client.

Supplies needed for clinician	**Supplies needed for client**
1. Handout	1. Handout

Instructions

1. Introduce the game to the client
2. Share your screen. This aids in visualization of game and client can also read prompts.
    a. Use writing tools on the application you are using to write in clients answers
    b. Or client can write in themselves

Useful websites, tools, resources or notes:

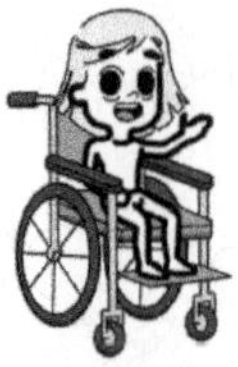

Positive Self-Talk

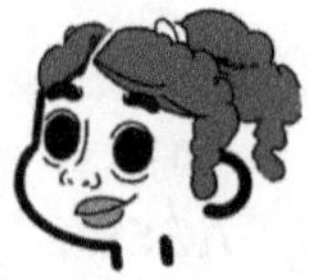

1) I felt good when...	2) I am proud of myself because....	3) I feel strong when .....
4) Something that when well today was....	5) I had fun when....	6) I learned from this mistake...
7) This was interesting today...	8) The best part of today...	9) A good quality I am learning today...
10) This makes me unique...	11) A way I was kind today was...	12) I like this about myself...
13) An accomplishment I made this week was...	14) I like this about myself...	15) Something I love about my life is...

ALL AGES

Finish the Sentence

Objectives

- Explore thoughts and feelings that may be affect client's self-esteem.
- Complete the worksheet at pre and post or at different times within the therapeutic relationship to gauge client's growth and internal processes.
- Assist as a conversation starter and relationship builder.

Supplies needed for clinician	**Supplies needed for client**
1. Handout	1. Handout 2. Pencil/Pen 3. Notepad to take notes if not using handout. 4. Dice

Instructions

- Enlarge the worksheet that you will be working on with client.
- Share on screen.
- You can use your apps writing tool to write in answers to question.
- The client can also write in answers in chat box.
- Take turns completing worksheet 1, 2 and 3.

Useful websites, tools, resources or notes:

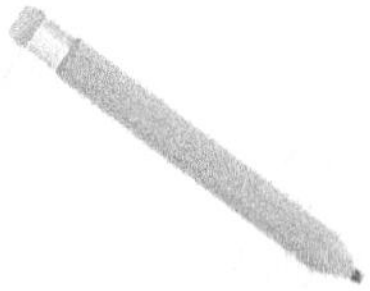

Finish the Sentence

Worksheet 1
1. The person I am closest to is
2. My one wish would
3. The scariest thing is
4. I am going to try to
5. I'd really enjoy
6. One goal I have for my future is
7. Someone who supports me is
Worksheet 2
1. I am happiest when
2. I was sad about
3. I love when
4. I hate when
5. I believe that
6. I was surprised to learn
7. My biggest fear is
Worksheet 3
1. Today is going to be
2. Today I struggled with
3. Today I will be kind with
4. Today I will try my best at
5. A funny thing that that happened today was

ALL AGES

Suitcase Termination Activity

Objectives:

- To role model healthy goodbyes.
- Help client identify and articulate feelings and thoughts regarding termination.
- To process what was gained in therapy; accomplishments, goals, coping skills, etc. . . Help prevent regression.

Supplies needed for clinician	**Supplies needed for client**
1. Handout	1. Handout 2. Paper, pencil, markers or colored pencils 3. Notepad to take notes if not using handout.

Instructions:

1. Provide the suitcase handout to client by email, text or share screen.
2. Ask them to write on their suitcase to answer this question.
    a. What have you learned in therapy? (coping skills, supports, accomplishments, resources etc.)
3. Process feelings about termination throughout the activity.

Useful websites, tools, resources or notes:

Suitcase Termination Activity

I wish you the best, Goodbye

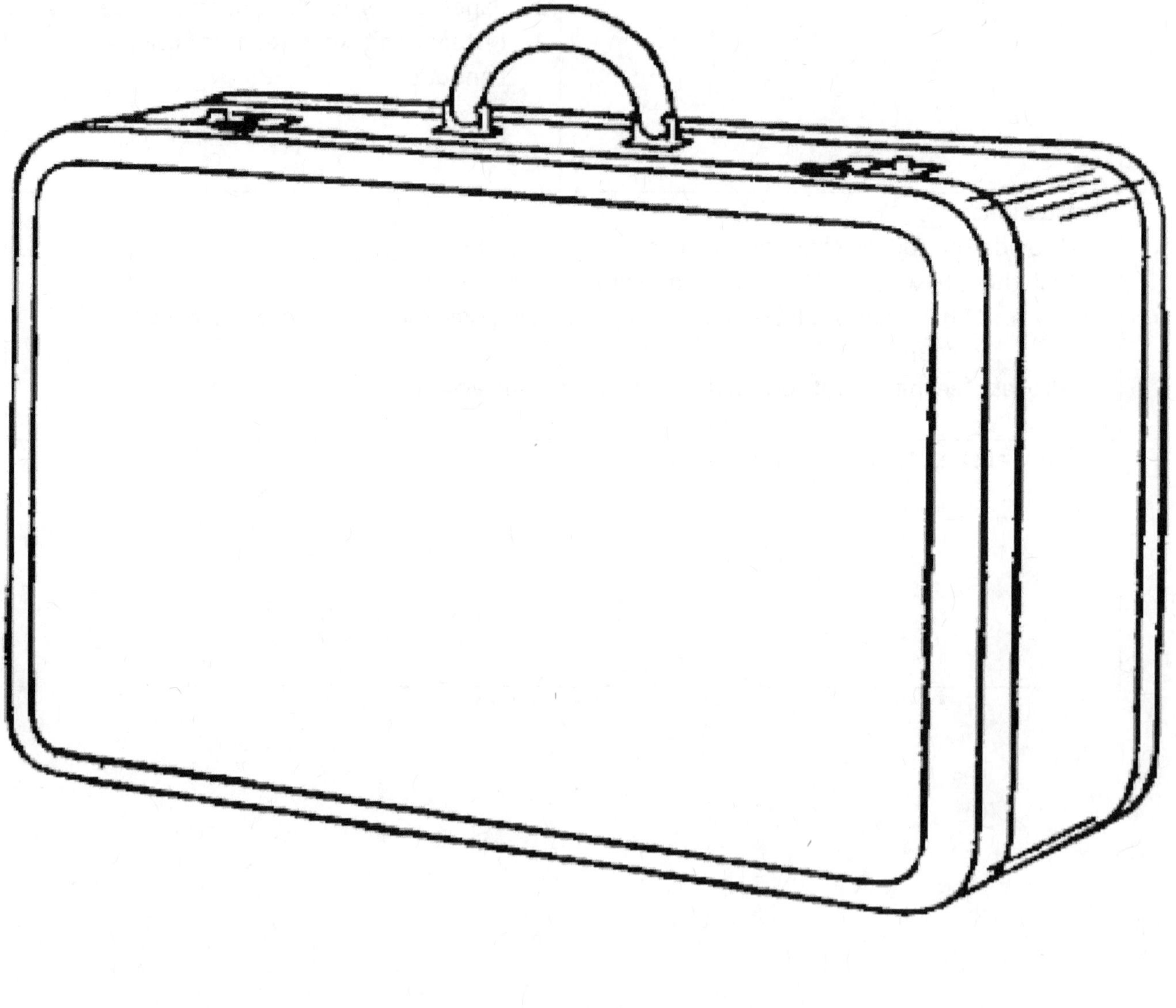

ALL AGES

Triggers, Cues, Behaviors

<table>
<tr><td colspan="2">Objectives
• To assist client in identifying triggers, cues and behaviors for their anger.
• Have client explore patterns to their behavior and replace with behaviors that are more positive.
• Build clients awareness of thoughts, behaviors and sensory responses.</td></tr>
<tr><td>Supplies needed for clinician
1. Handout
2. Dice</td><td>Supplies needed for client
1. Handout
2. Pencil/Pen
3. Notepad to take notes if not using handout.
4. Dice</td></tr>
<tr><td colspan="2">Instructions:
1. Clinician to introduce the game to the client and share on teleconference screen. This aid in visualization of game and client can also read prompts. 2.
2. Use writing tool on teleconference application and write in clients answers and /or depending on client's age, have them write in chat box.</td></tr>
<tr><td colspan="2">Useful websites, tools, or resources:</td></tr>
</table>

Triggers, Cues, Behaviors

TRIGGERS (What happens right before I get angry?)	CUES (Where do I feel anger in my body)	BEHAVIORS (what do I do after I become angry? What do I do?)

ALL AGES

What Leads to Anger

Objectives

- Explore triggers and antecedents to anger.
- Assist client with identifying feelings that lead to anger.
- Discover and address patterns of client's behavior.

Supplies needed for clinician	**Supplies needed for client**
1. Handout	1. Handout 2. Pencil/Pen 3. Notepad to take notes if not using handout.

Instructions:

1. Introduce the game to the client and share on your screen.
2. This aids in visualization of game and client can also read prompts.
3. Use writing tool on app to write in clients answers and /or depending on clients age, have them write in chat box.

Useful websites, tools, resources or notes:

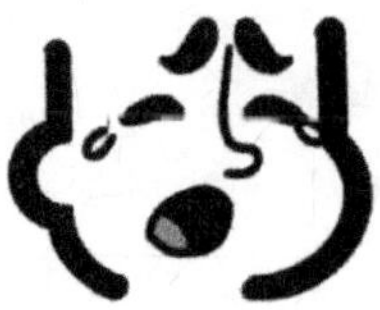

What Leads to Anger?

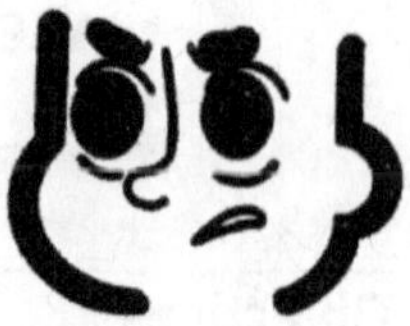

Sometimes people become angry when they feel sad, ignored, embarrassed, or frustrated.

What makes you feel sad?

____

____

____

What makes you feel ignored?

____

____

____

What makes you feel embarrassed?

____

____

____

What makes you feel frustrated?

____

____

____

Do any of you answers match your "anger triggers"?
Which ones:

____

____

____

ALL AGES

You Tube Videos

(No Handout Needed)

Objectives

- To explain and help client understand abstract and difficult topics for younger audiences.
- To identify and articulate feelings and thoughts.

Supplies needed for clinician	Supplies needed for client
1. Handout	1. Handout

Instructions

1. Choose a video that is relevant to concern affecting child.
2. Share on screen. Practice display and sound beforehand.
3. Allow time for processing video afterwards.
4. Have child state what stood out for them, what they will remember, what they liked or did not like.

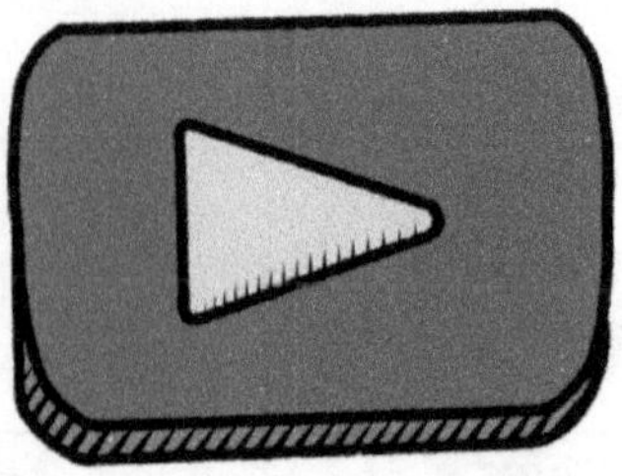

YouTube Links

- Preschool – 8
    - A story about social distancing: https://www.youtube.com/watch?v=DA_SsZFYw0w
- K-8
    - Howard Wiggle Bottoms story about managing his anger: https://www.youtube.com/watch?v=2IqVJHVkTLE
    - Howard Wiggle Bottom story about doing your best: https://www.youtube.com/watch?v=haChyOmVQas
- K- 12
    - The Present, a story about remaining positive: https://www.youtube.com/watch?v=WjqiU5FgsYc
- K-3
    - Guess and Learn about Emotions: https://youtu.be/iKMFKiTaF5s
    - PBS: https://www.youtube.com/watch?v=37w9JjUWN30https://pbskids.org/daniel/games/guess-the-feeling
- K-12.
    - Anxiety Explained https://www.youtube.com/watch?v=rpolpKTWrp4&list=PLehGvMkd5jMbl8csm0WqOKBBJFT3DN5DA&index=22&t=53s
- K- 3
    - Story about grief and loss : https://www.youtube.com/watch?v=QdYCsxC8EHY
- K-Adult
    - 3 minute mindfulness https://www.youtube.com/watch?v=ihwcw_ofuME

- K-5
    - 2 minute mindfulness- Breathing Butterfly https://www.youtube.com/watch?v=FxHTbLZ66JY

More meditations

- https://www.innerhealthstudio.com/relaxation-scripts-for-children.html
- https://self-compassion.org/category/exercises/?fbclid=IwAR05agNdFq6sWZeGDslPE6O7xKmtFaDpbXs1Td-kaDBb3gaT27g6cU371qo

ALL AGES

Vision Board

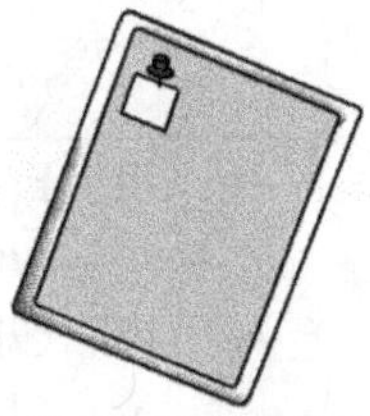

Objectives

- Articulate an achievement goal and identifying behaviors needed to get there.
- Help client identify dreams and behaviors needed to get there.

Supplies needed for clinician	**Supplies needed for client**
1. Handout 2. Pinterest Account	1. Handout 2. Pinterest Account

Instructions

- Introduce the idea of "vision boards" to the client
- Share screen, email or text client.
- STEP 1: Make a list of 3-4 goals that you want on your vision board
    a. Some questions to consider
        i. If you could be, do, or have anything, what would it be?
        ii. What do you dream about (places, books, songs, movies, favorite animals, etc)?
        iii. Who do you look up to?
- Log on to Pinterest to create an account.
    a. Click your profile picture to open your profile and then click the plus icon at the top of the page
    b. Click Create board
    c. Enter a name for your board and click the box next to "Visibility" if you want to keep this board secret
    d. Click into the field beside "Add dates" to add a start and end date
    e. Click Create
- STEP 2: Search for photos of the 3-4 goals together or assign for homework
    a. Travel, Health, Career, Family, Love Friendship, Experiences, Role models
- STEP 3: Search for photos together or assign for homework of ways to achieve goals.
    a. For example: If goal is to become a doctor, look for pictures of college, studying, going to school. If goal is to become a professional basketball player, look for pictures of going to practice, learning about kinesiology or studying to stay on the school basketball team.
    b. Create a SECTION for each goal
        i. Click your profile picture to open your profile and then click the plus icon at the top of the page
        ii. Click Create board

iii. Enter a name for your board and click the box next to "Visibility" if you want to keep this board secret iv. Click into the field beside "Add dates" to add a start and end date v. Click Create
Useful websites, tools, resources or notes: Website: https://help.pinterest.com/en Notes: • Processing can occur at every step of this activity. • Activity can spread across several sessions.

ALL AGES

Feeling Word Clouds for Individual or Groups

Objectives

- To help clients articulate emotions, ideas or thoughts.
- To engage clients in a grounding activity linked to the topic of the session.

Supplies needed for clinician

1. Handout
2. Mentimeter account

Supplies needed for client

1. Handout
2. Website address and code for activity

Instructions

1. Setup needed before session
   a. This is how you create a Word Cloud with Mentimeter:
      i. Sign up for an account
      ii. Click on Create a new slide
      iii. Click Choose Word Cloud
      iv. Fill in your question: ex. Name 3 emotions that you have felt this week.
      v. The website will produce a code for you to share with your clients.
2. Introduce the idea of "Word Clouds" to the clients in your group
3. Share screen, email or text client the instructions that state: "Go to menti.com and use the code ####".

Group: Send code to group to create a Word Cloud for the group session

Individual: Send the code and ask client to answer the question every day for 1 week to create a word cloud.

Useful websites, tools, resources or notes:

Website: https://www.mentimeter.com/app

SAMPLE

What are some of the emotions that you have felt this week? list up to 3

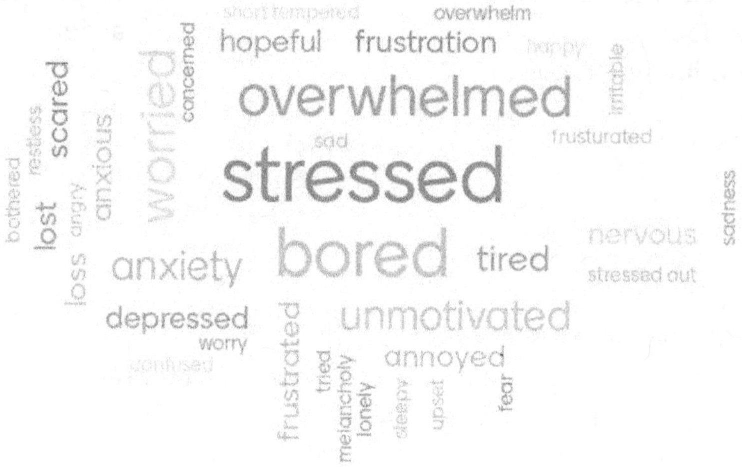

ALL AGES

Glass House

Objectives

- Understanding family dynamics.

Supplies needed for clinician

1. Handout

Supplies needed for client

1. Handout
2. Pen, pencil, marker, color pencil or crayon.

Instructions

1. Provide handouts to the client(s) via text, email, or Google Docs.
2. Ask the client(s) to list under each category.
3. Guide the client(s) through the activity by asking relevant questions in order to better understand the client and their family dynamic.

Useful websites, tools, resources or notes:

Glass House

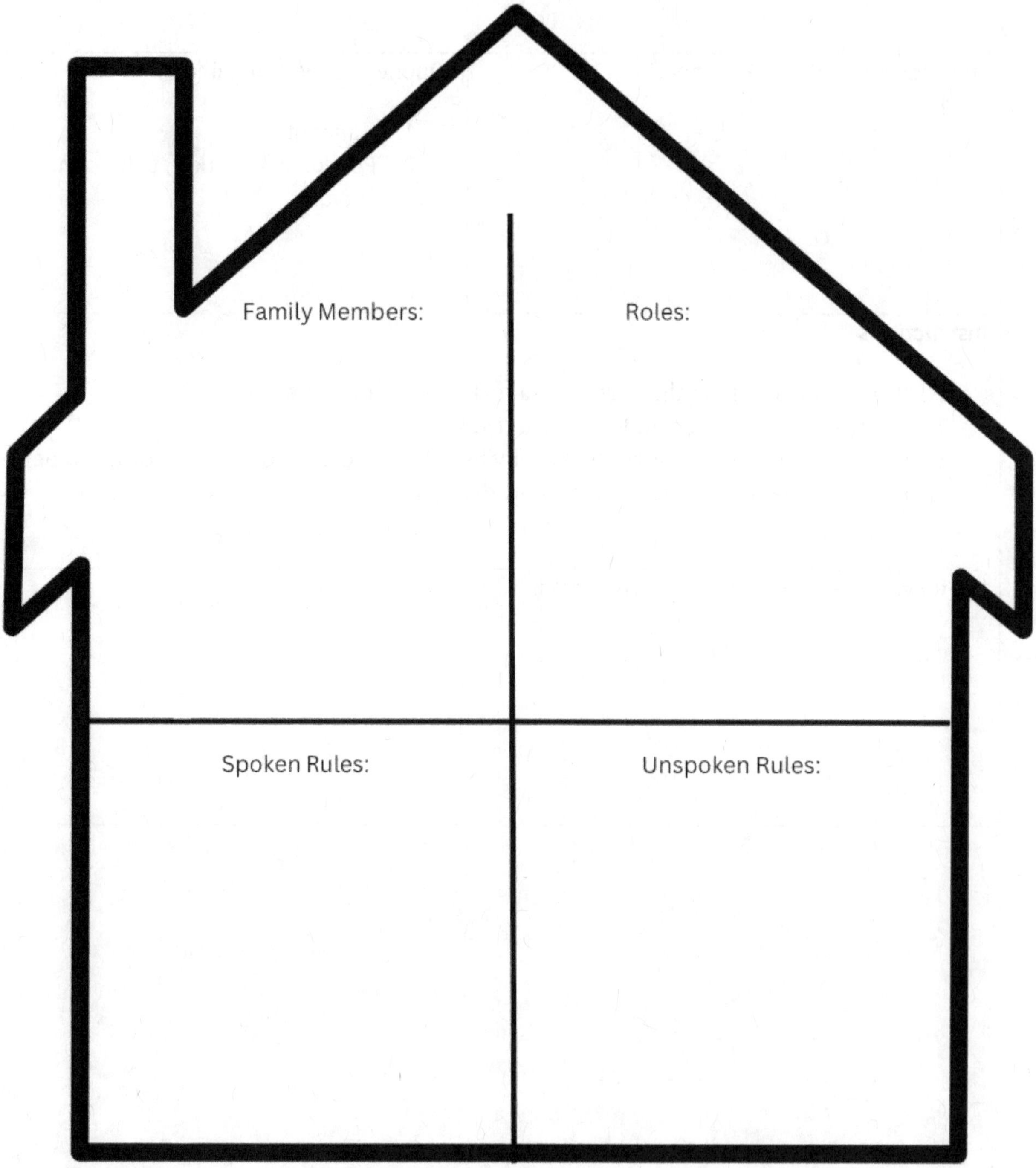

ALL AGES

Genogram

Objectives	
Record and interpret family history to better understand the genetic, medical, social, and cultural aspects of the client's family.	
Supplies needed for clinician 2. Handout	**Supplies needed for client** 3. Handout 4. Pen, pencil, marker, color pencil or crayon.
Instructions 1. Start with the client(s) and draw a square or circle to represent your gender. Connect the client to their parents and siblings with vertical lines. Add the clients' grandparents by drawing horizontal lines connecting them to your parents. Continue this process to represent multiple generations. 2. Use the key provided.	
Useful websites, tools, resources or notes: Website: https://genopro.com/genogram/rules/	

Genogram

Key:

ALL AGES

Proof is in the Pudding

Objectives

Building on clients' self-esteem by identifying the clients' strengths and successful past experiences.

Supplies needed for clinician

1. Handout

Supplies needed for client

1. Handout
2. Pen, pencil, markers, highlighters, color pencils, or crayons.
3. magazines
4. scissors
5. Glue

Instructions

1. Have the client list the things they love about themselves internally and externally.
2. Have the client cut images out of magazines to represent the things they love/like about themselves.
3. Have the client glue the cut outs onto the handout provided by the clinician.

Useful websites, tools, resources or notes:

Website:

Proof is in the Pudding

Adolescent

Double Sided Mirror

Objectives

To improve cultural sensitivity and treatment by focusing clinical attention on the patient's perspective and social context.

Supplies needed for clinician

1. Handout

Supplies needed for client

1. Handout
2. Pen, pencil, maker, color pencil or crayon.

Instructions

1. Have the client list the things they love about themselves internally and externally.
2. Have the client cut images out of magazines to represent the things they love/like about themselves.
3. Have the client glue the cut outs onto the handout provided by the clinician.

Useful websites, tools, resources or notes:

Website:

Double Sided Mirror

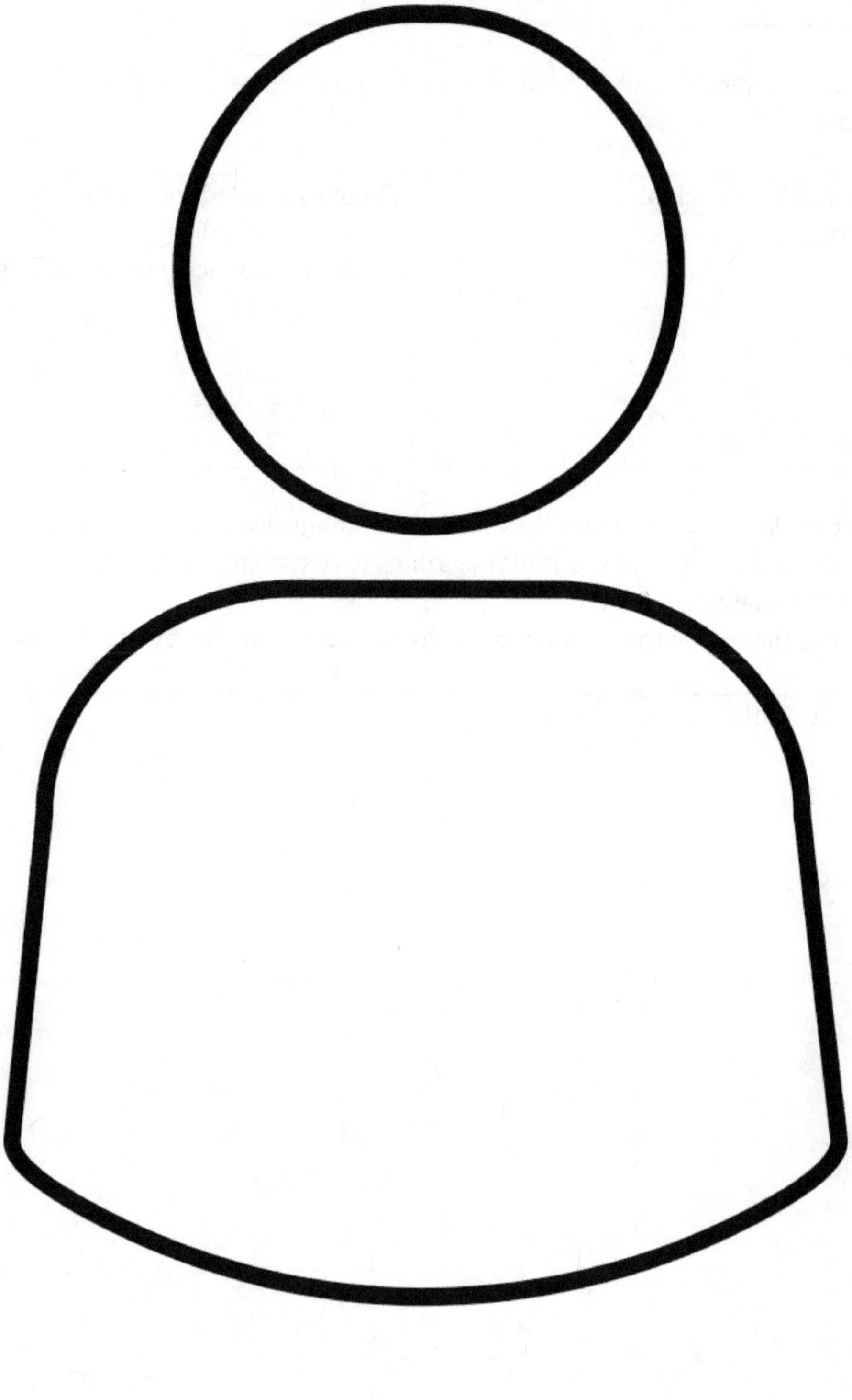

ALL AGES

Reading Between the Lines

Objectives

- Help the client identify unspoken communication through body language and facial expressions.

Supplies needed for clinician	**Supplies needed for client**
1. Instructions of the Handout	

Instructions

1. Have the client provide a scenario from their personal experience.
2. Act out scenarios and have client(s) interpret the nonverbal cues.
3. The clinician can provide scenarios of their own or emotions based on the clients' needs.

Useful websites, tools, resources or notes:

Website:

ALL AGES

Circle of Control

Objectives	
• Activity for helping clients cope with anxiety and depression by building coping skills.	
Supplies needed for clinician 1. Handout	**Supplies needed for client** 1. Handout 2. Pen, pencil, maker, color pencil or crayon.
Instructions 1. Provide the client with psycho-education on anxiety and depression. 2. Ask the client about their idea of coping with anxiety and depression. 3. Use the handout to work with the client on identifying what are some of the factors they are able to control internally and externally.	
Useful websites, tools, resources or notes: Website:	

Circle of Control

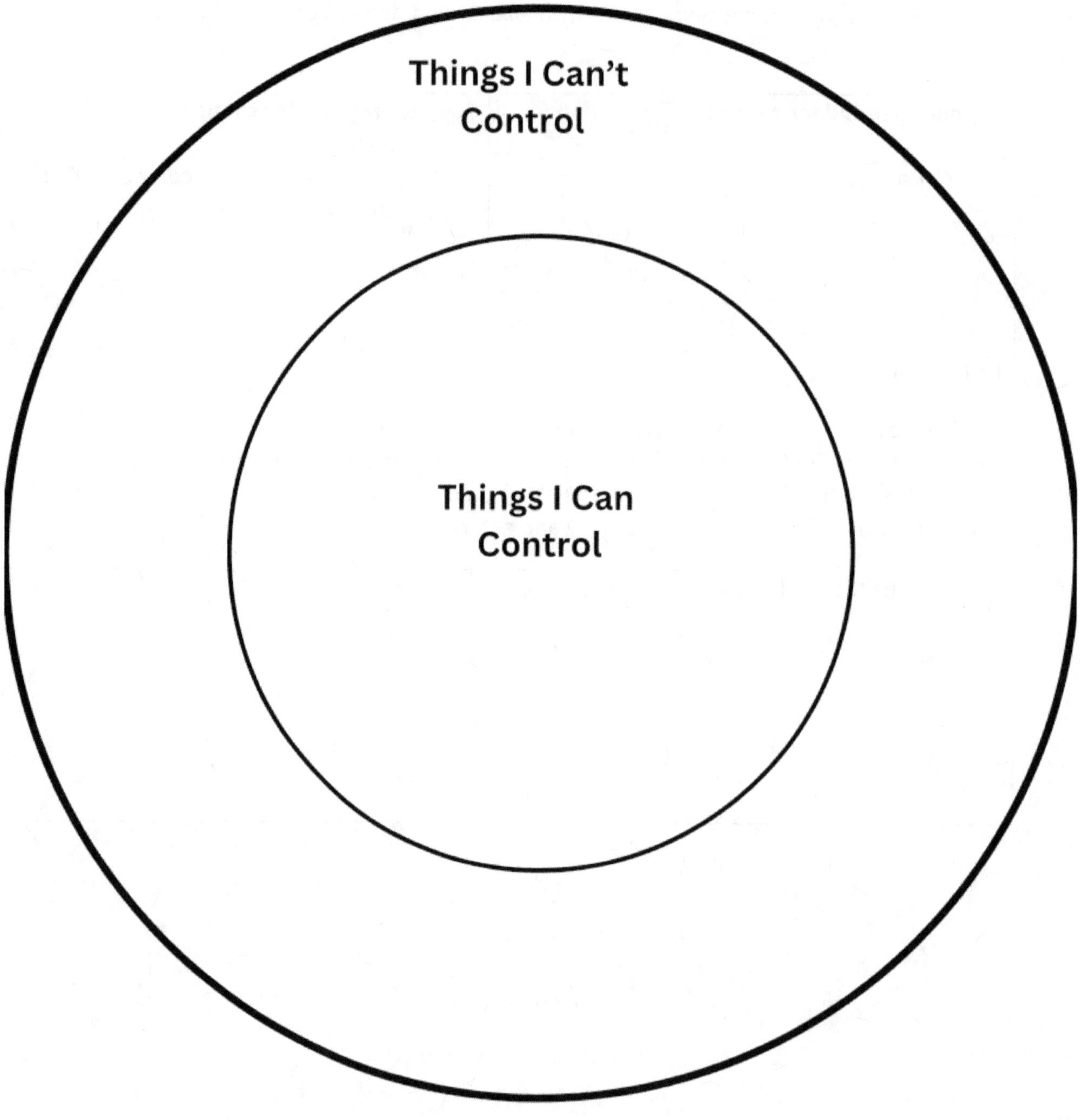

ALL AGES

Caring for a Broken Heart

Objectives
Activity for coping with grief and loss of all kinds.

Supplies needed for clinician	**Supplies needed for client**
1. Handout	1. Handout/red cardstock 2. Scissors 3. band-aids 4. pencil, markers, crayons, pens, etc

Instructions

1. Have the client cut out a heart on red cardstock paper.
2. Have the client write down specific things, people, and/or memories that he/she is experiencing.
3. Rip the heart into smaller pieces so that each piece has a 'loss' on it.
4. Pull band-aids and use them to tape the pieces of the heart back together and write a strength that helps the client cope with the situation.

Useful websites, tools, resources or notes:

Website: empoweremotions.com

Caring for a Broken Heart

ALL AGES

Pieces of the "Bye"

Objectives

- Activity for coping with grief and loss of all kinds. This activity is intended to empower clients about the narrative behind a loss.

Supplies needed for clinician	**Supplies needed for client**
1. Handout	1. Handout 2. Pen, pencil, maker, color pencil or crayon.

Instructions

1. Provide the client with psycho-education about grief and loss.
2. Review and fill out the different open fields with the client.

Useful websites, tools, resources or notes:

Website:

Pieces of the "Bye"

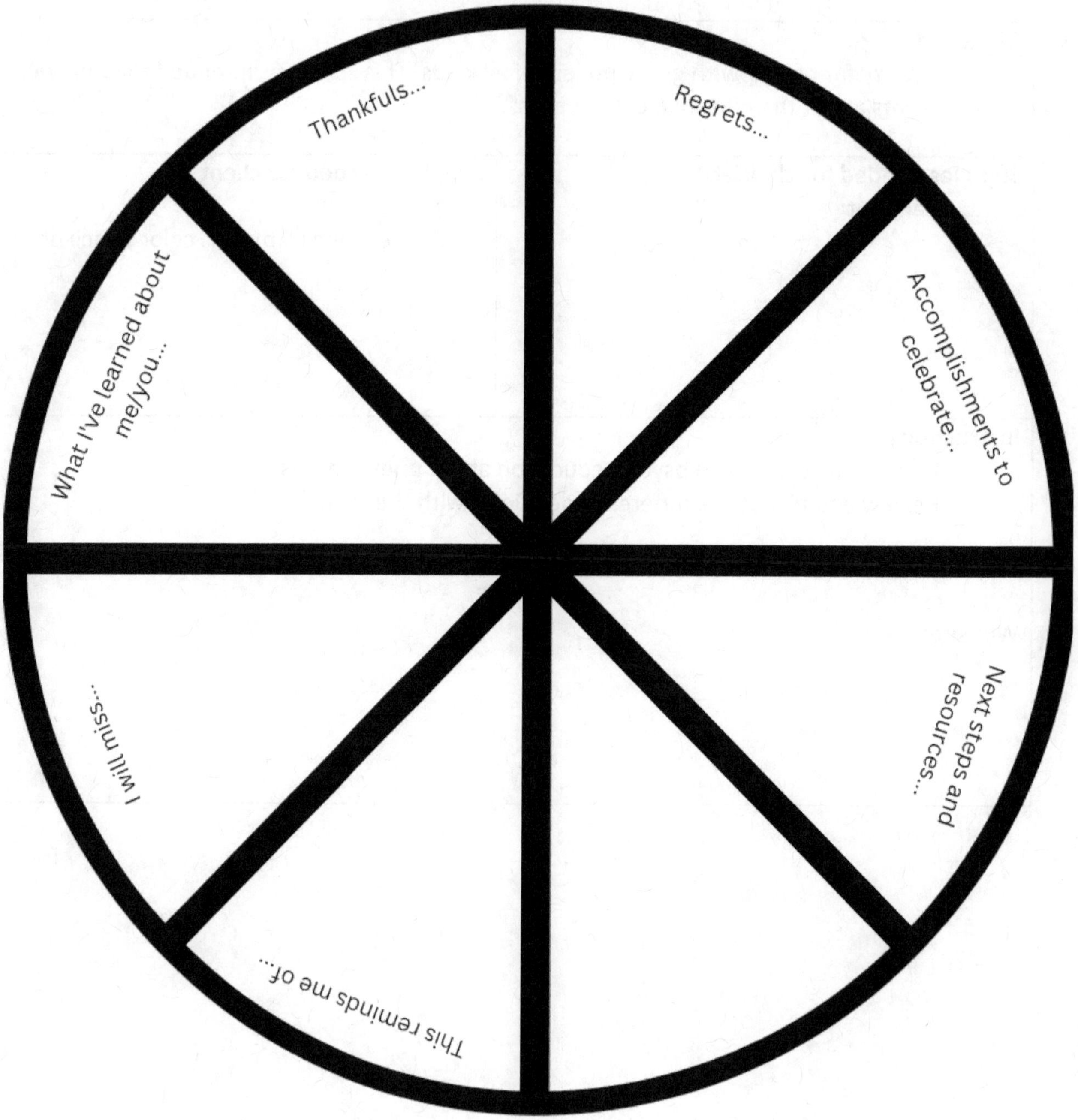

Children

If I Didn’t Care

Adolescents

Objectives

Activity to help clients build self-esteem and character building.

Supplies needed for clinician	**Supplies needed for client**
1. Handout	1. Handout 2. Pen, pencil, maker, color pencil or crayon.

Instructions

1. Provide psycho-education about anxiety and depression.
2. Discuss different scenarios where the client explores a judgment-free life.
3. fill out the fields with the client.

Useful websites, tools, resources or notes:

Website:

If I Didn't Care

If you didn't care what other people thought or said about you, what are some things you would do differently than you are doing now?

I would ______________________________

I would not______________________________

I would say______________________________

I would listen to ______________________________

I would start ______________________________

I would go ______________________________

I would try ______________________________

I would watch ______________________________

I would stop ______________________________

I would no longer ______________________________

Color My Mood

Objectives Mood check to identify the range of moods a client may feel at once.	
Supplies needed for clinician 2. Handout	**Supplies needed for client** 3. Handout 4. Pen, pencil, maker, color pencil or crayon.
Instructions 1. Provide psych-education on emotions. 2. validate client's different emotions 3. Have client associate colors to an emotion(s) by filling out the key. 4. have client color in the outline with the colors of feelings they are feeling during session/ event.	
Useful websites, tools, resources or notes: Website:	

Color My Mood

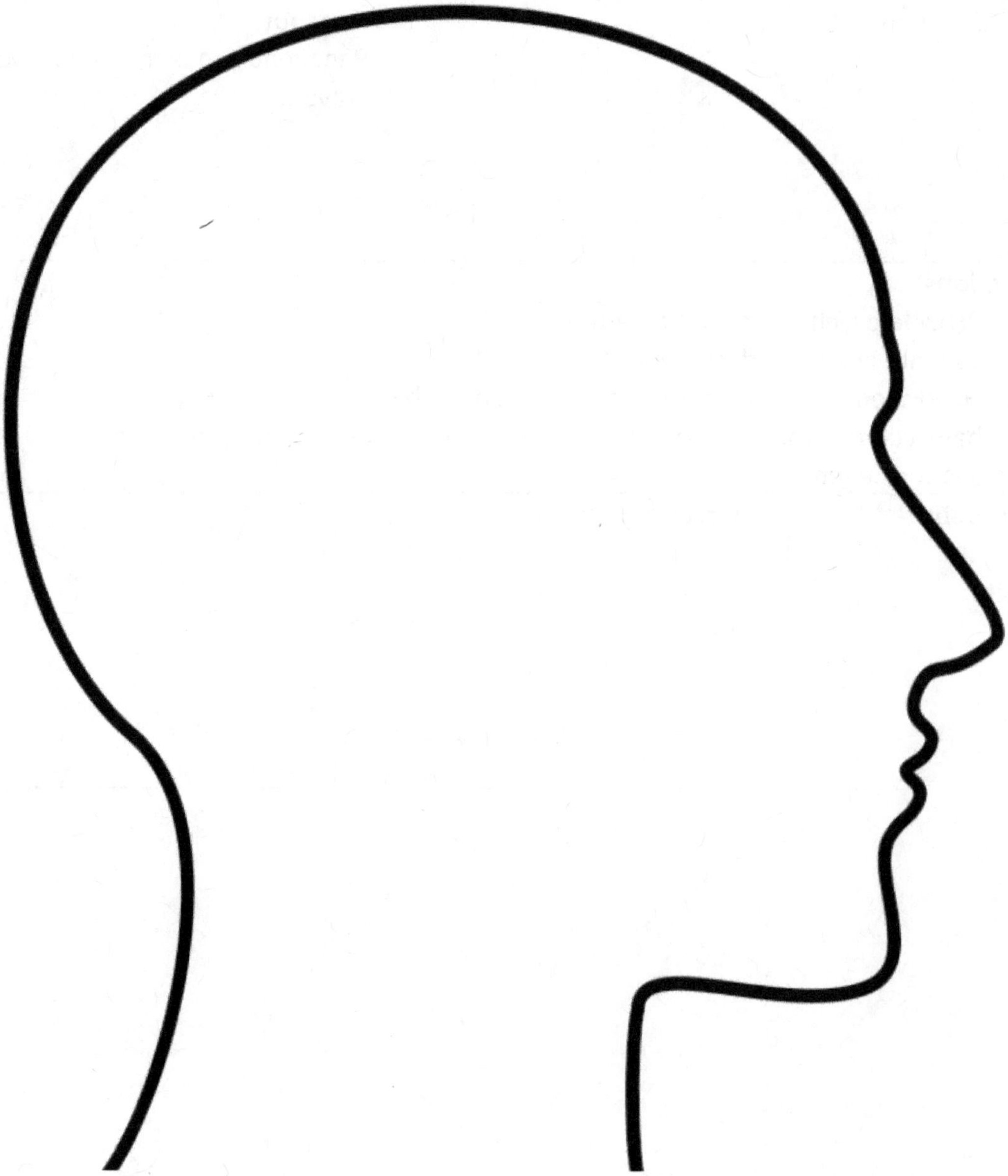

Appendices

Appendix A

How to use technology to fluidly respond to the emotions of another person

Therapeutic Rapport: Research shows that this a strong predictor of treatment response in mental health settings. It is defined as the working relationship between the mental health clinician and patient and includes shared goals for treatment, the presence of warmth, authenticity, genuine concern, and a collaborative bond (Lopez, 2019).

Figure 1 Establishing Therapeutic Rapport in Telebehavioral Health

Technology

Adequate Bandwith

- Helps improve video images to appreciate affect, body movements, eye contact, gestures
- Prevents time lapse in verbal transmission to approximate in person sessions
- Benefits appreciation of subtle changes in facial expression, blunting, quivering, aids in detecting tremor in anxiety etc.

Camera Placement

- Adequate lighting is important for clinician and client
- Ask to be able to see at least upper half of clients body
- Ask all participants to be fully visible in camera or have them each sign on with own phone or computer.

Microphones

- Insist for client to wear earphones or some kind of headset to be able to clearly detect the patients speech and preserve a confidential working space.

Backup Systems

- Have a plan if a session is disconnected due to a system failure.
- Phone or computer

Picture in Picture

- Helps you monitor your own facial expression to help you with feedback and self-monitor your own expressions.
- You don't have this immediate feedback in face to face sessions. Use it.
- Move your picture and your clients picture right under the camera on your computer or on your phone so that you look like you have eye contact with you clients.
- Eye contact has been found to be essential in establishing therapeutic rapport.

Interventions

Offer a Practice Session

- Allow time to practice with your client to log on, learning the program and to ask questions

Explain Telebehavioral Health to your clients

- Some research shows that they are more comfortable with it than the clinician.
- Explore their comfort or discomfort on an ongoing basis.
- Explain the risks and the benefits
- Explore your client's past experience with telehealth in any setting
- Tell them why it's being used

Workspace

- Sitting- Sit at a desk or table that allows you free movement to access online or computer resources or so that your client is able to see at least the upper half of your body. Avoid sitting on beds, couches or floors.
- Set up a designated area that approximates a clinical setting. Clients are able to see your background. Choose your background very thoughtfully. Ex. Library, blank wall, office

Professional Presence

- Use of professional self- You may be working from home but you should show up to session in professional dress that is expected of your worksite.

Engagement

- Look into camera
- Speak up
- Speak clearly
- Be gentle
- Be mindful of your comfort and discomfort

Appendix B

Apps for Online Document Annotation and Markup Tools

What are online document annotation and markup tools?

- Online document annotation and markup tools help you collaborate with your clients when they don't have access to paper, pens, crayons or other art supplies. These apps help you and your client highlight, underline, and strikethrough text in PDF and other document formats. It is an assistive technology tool that can help students with special needs participate in activities with you. You can add text boxes, shapes, and images. You can easily collaborate on documents while in session and avoid the hassles of printing documents.

What does "Apps" mean?

- The word is short for "application." Application refers to a software application for a phone or a computer. They are designed to run on a mobile device such as a phone, notebook, computer, or watch. In our case we use these apps to allow us to perform specific educational and therapeutic tasks.

List of apps to consider:

- Google for Education- https://edu.google.com/?modal_active=none
- Kami: https://www.kamiapp.com/?ref=producthunt
- PDF Annotator: https://www.pdfannotator.com/en/
- Diigo: https://www.diigo.com
- Bounce: https://bounceapp.com

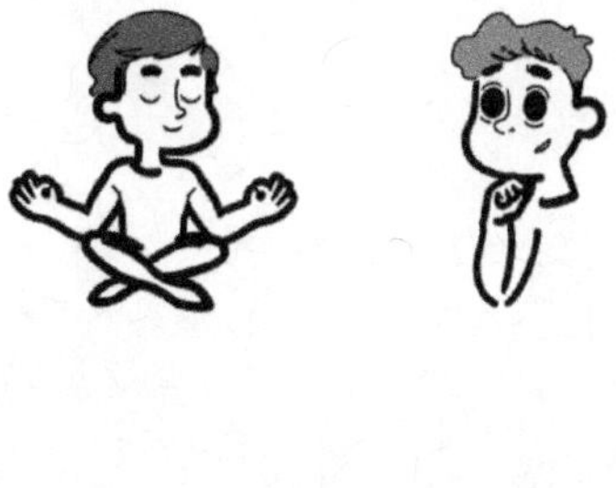

Appendix C

10 HIPPAA Compliant Technology Platforms

HIPAA (Health Insurance Portability and Accountability Act) guidelines require mental health providers who transmit electronic PHI (Protected Health Information), to adopt privacy and security safeguards. The following are 10 platforms that are HIPAA compliant. They are listed in alphabetical order. It is up to each mental health provider to research which technology platform suits them best. This listing is not be considered as an endorsement of any of the products. We are simply listing them to help you begin your search for HIPAA compliant platforms.

1. Doxy.me: https://doxy.me
2. TheraLINK: https://www.thera-link.com
3. Theranest: https://theranest.com
4. Zoom for Healthcare: https://zoom.us/healthcare
5. GoToMeeting: https://www.gotomeeting.com
6. Medici: https://www.medici.md
7. Vsee: https://vsee.com
8. Simple Practice: https://www.simplepractice.com
9. Ring Central for Healthcare: https://www.ringcentral.com
10. VTConnect: https://vtconnect.net

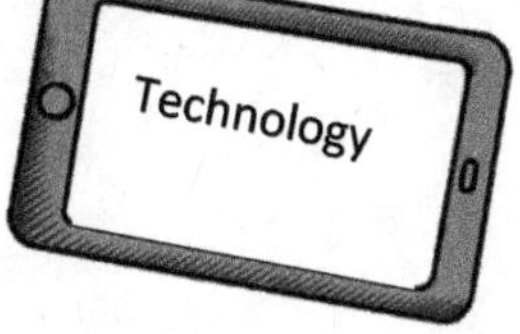

Appendix D

Online Assessment Tools

Online assessment tools are helpful in telemental health work. The following are links to websites that provide free online assessment tools. Use your professional judgement when choosing which tools are best for you client.

- **DSM V Online Assessment Measures:** "These patient assessment measures were developed to be administered at the initial patient interview and to monitor treatment progress, thus serving to advance the use of initial symptomatic status and patient reported outcome (PRO) information, as well as the use of "anchored" severity assessment instruments" (*Diagnostic and statistical manual of mental disorders: DSM-52013*)
  - https://www.psychiatry.org/psychiatrists/practice/dsm/educational-resources/assessment-measures
- **MDCALC:** PHQ9 for Depression, GAD 7 for Anxiety, Hamilton Anxiety Scale, Columbia Suicide Severity Scale...etc.
  - https://www.mdcalc.com
- **Mental Health America:** screening available for Depression Test, Postpartum Depression Test, Anxiety Test, Psychosis Test, Bipolar Test, Eating Disorder Test, PTSD Test, Parent Test, Youth Test, Addiction Test, Prueba De Depresión (Depression Test - Spanish), Prueba De Ansiedad (Anxiety Test - Spanish), Better Care For Adults, Work Health Survey, Healthcare Worker Survey ...etc.
  - https://screening.mhanational.org/screening-tools
- **Psycom:** Depression, Bipolar Disorder, Obsessive-Compulsive Disorder (OCD), Generalized Anxiety Disorder (GAD), Schizophrenia, Mania, Bulimia, Borderline Personality Disorder (BPD), Sexual Addiction...etc.
  - https://www.psycom.net

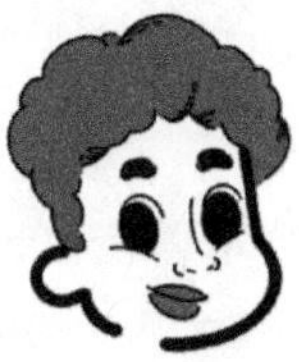

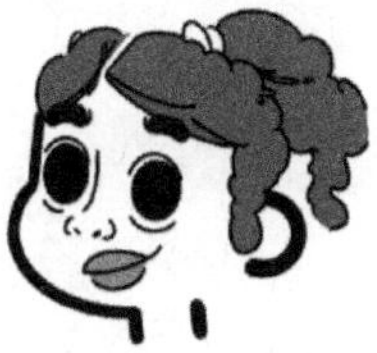

Biographies

Flor Chaidez PPSC, LCSW is a licensed clinical social worker with 20+ years of experience working in School Mental Health in local school districts. She has a private practice and continues to train Social Work interns. Flor Chaidez was raised in North East Los Angeles. This experience has informed her view on working on social justice and mental health issues. Shelter-in-place made her realize that mental health providers were lacking tools, as we all were adapting to a new normal. https://www.chaidezsupportservices.com/

Obregon Psychological & Educational Services

Verónica Obregón, PPSC, LCSW, Ed.D. is a licensed clinical social worker with 20+ years of School Mental Health experience. She is a full-time Adjunct at a local university teaching for the MSW and BSW programs. She has a hybrid private practice providing individual psychotherapy and mental health consultation to organizations. Dr. Obregon was born in Mexico City and raised in East Los Angeles. Her origins have always fueled her drive for social justice and mental health. www.veronicaobregon.com

End User License Agreement

AKA One User License Agreement

TERMS OF USE

You bought a **one**-user license agreement for this product. That means that this product is for your use only and may not be copied to share with another person. If another person asks you to share or copy this item, it is only ethical for you to direct them to the location where you purchased this item.

YOU MAY USE

- For personal use
- To use with clients

DO NOT

- Give this to others
- Copy this book or any part of this book for use by others
- Post this book or any part of this book on a public or searchable website
- Copy or modify this book for sale

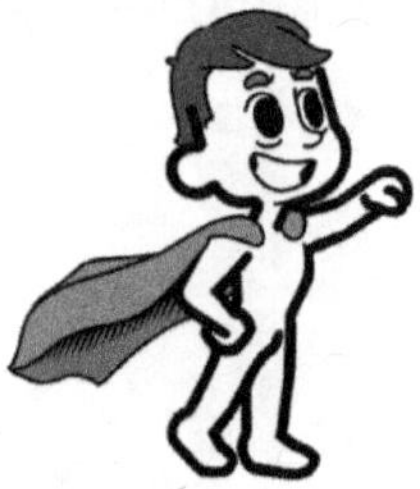

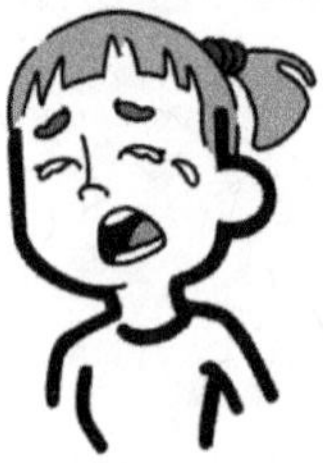

References

Augusterfer, E., Mollica, R., & Lavelle, J. (2015). *A review of telemental health in international and post-disaster settings* doi:10.3109/09540261.2015.1082985

Augusterfer, E., Mollica, R., & Lavelle, J. (2018). Leveraging technology in post-disaster settings: The role of digital health/telemental health. *Current Psychiatry Reports, 20*(10), 1-8. doi:10.1007/s11920-018-0953-4

Brunzell, T., Stokes, H., & Waters, L. (2016). Trauma-informed positive education: Using positive psychology to strengthen vulnerable students. *Contemporary School Psychology, 20*(1), 63-83. doi:10.1007/s40688-015-0070-x

Clark, R. E. (2008). *Turning research into results : A guide to selecting the right performance solutions*. Charlotte, NC: Information Age Publishing Inc. Retrieved from /z-wcorg/

Contreras, S., Porras-Javier, L., Zima, B., Soares, N., Park, C., Patel, A., et al. (2018). Development of a telehealth-coordinated intervention to improve access to community-based mental health. *Ethnicity & Disease, 28*, 457-466. doi:10.18865/ed.28.S2.457

Glueck, D. (2013). *3 - establishing therapeutic rapport in telemental health* Elsevier Inc. doi:10.1016/B978-0-12-416048-4.00003-8

Goldstein, F., & Glueck, D. (2016). Developing rapport and therapeutic alliance during telemental health sessions with children and adolescents. *Journal of Child and Adolescent Psychopharmacology, 26*(3), 24-211. doi:10.1089/cap.2015.0022

Grady, B., Myers, K. M., Nelson, E., Belz, N., Bennett, L., Carnahan, L., et al. (2011). Evidence-based practice for telemental health. *Telemedicine Journal and E-Health, 17*(2), 131-148. doi:10.1089/tmj.2010.0158

Hassija, C., & Gray, M. J. (2011). The effectiveness and feasibility of videoconferencing technology to provide evidence-based treatment to rural domestic violence and sexual assault populations. *Telemedicine Journal and E-Health, 17*(4), 39-315. doi:10.1089/tmj.2010.0147

Hilty, D. M., Ferrer, D. C., Parish, M. B., Johnston, B., Callahan, E. J., & Yellowlees, P. M. (2013). The effectiveness of telemental health: A 2013 review. *Telemedicine Journal and E-Health, 19*(6), 444-454. doi:10.1089/tmj.2013.0075

Jones, A. M., Shealy, K. M., Reid-Quiñones, K., Moreland, A. D., Davidson, T. M., López, C. M., et al. (2014). Guidelines for establishing a telemental health program to provide evidence-based therapy for trauma-exposed children and families. *Psychological Services, 11*(4), 398-409. doi:10.1037/a0034963

Lambert, M. J., & Barley, D. E. (2001). Research summary on the therapeutic relationship and psychotherapy outcome. *Psychotherapy: Theory, Research, Practice, Training, 38*(4), 357-361. doi:10.1037/0033-3204.38.4.357

Lopez, A., Schwenk, S., Schneck, C. D., Griffin, R. J., & Mishkind, M. C. (2019). Technology-based mental health treatment and the impact on the therapeutic alliance. *Current Psychiatry Reports, 21*(8), 1-7. doi:10.1007/s11920-019-1055-7

Lipschitz, J. M., Connolly, S. L., Van Boxtel, R., Potter, J. R., Nixon, N., & Bidargaddi, N. (2023). Provider Perspectives on Telemental Health Implementation: Lessons Learned During the COVID-19 Pandemic and Paths Forward. Psychological Services, 20, 11-19. 10.1037/ser0000625

Myers, K., & Comer, J. (2016). The case for telemental health for improving the accessibility and quality of children's mental health services. *Journal of Child and Adolescent Psychopharmacology, 26*(3), 186-191. doi:10.1089/cap.2015.0055

Revere, D., Nelson, K., Thiede, H., Duchin, J., Stergachis, A., & Baseman, J. (2011). Public health emergency preparedness and response communications with health care providers: A literature review.(research article). *BMC Public Health, 11*, 337.

Stamoulos, C., Trepanier, L., Bourkas, S., Bradley, S., Stelmaszczyk, K., Schwartzman, D., et al. (2016). Psychologists' perceptions of the importance of common factors in psychotherapy for successful treatment outcomes. *Journal of Psychotherapy Integration, 26*(3), 300-317. doi:10.1037/a0040426

Stewart, R. W., Orengo-Aguayo, R., Cohen, J. A., Mannarino, A. P., & de Arellano, M.,A. (2017). A pilot study of trauma-focused Cognitive–Behavioral therapy delivered via telehealth technology. *Child Maltreatment, 22*(4), 324-333. doi:10.1177/1077559517725403

Stewart, R. W., Orengo-Aguayo, R., Wallace, M., Metzger, I. W., & Rheingold, A. A. (2019). Leveraging technology and cultural adaptations to increase access and engagement among trauma-exposed african american youth: Exploratory study of school-based telehealth delivery of trauma-focused cognitive behavioral therapy. *Journal of Interpersonal Violence,* , 886260519831380.

Ulzen, T., Williamson, L., Foster, P., & Parris-Barnes, K. (2013). The evolution of a community-based telepsychiatry program in rural alabama: Lessons learned--A brief report. *Community Mental Health Journal, 49*(1), 101-5. doi:10.1007/s10597-012-9493-2

Worldometers.info. *Worldometer.* Retrieved June 5, 2020, from https://www.worldometers.info/coronavirus/country/us/

www.ingramcontent.com/pod-product-compliance
Lightning Source LLC
LaVergne TN
LVHW060453061126
851857LV00016B/1811
* 9 7 9 8 3 8 5 1 6 2 1 8 5 *